Lou Gehrig Disease, ALS or Amyotrophic Lateral
Sclerosis explained.

ALS symptoms, signs, stages, types, diagnosis,
treatment, caregiver tips, aids and what to expect is all
covered.

by

Robert Rymore

Published by IMB Publishing 2013

Table of Contents

Table of Contents

Table of Contents

Acknowledgements

I would like to thank all of the organizations who made this book possible, including The ALS Association, The Muscular Dystrophy Association, Massachusetts General Hospital, The National Institutes of Health, The Mayo Clinic, Emory University, and Harvard Medical School.

Foreword

Several years ago, when my childhood friend was diagnosed with Lou Gehrig's Disease, or ALS, I knew very little about the disease. As my friend and her family reeled from her diagnosis, I did what I always do when confronting the unknown. I started researching. I really wanted to know more about Lou Gehrig's Disease, how it would affect my friend, what kind of treatment is typically used to treat it, and how I could help her and her family in the upcoming years.

I struggled to find a comprehensive book that answered my questions in a straightforward, easy-to-understand manner. Most of the books were filled with medical jargon that really made learning a challenge and left me with more questions.

The more I looked, the more frustrated I became. I decided I would start talking to professionals – doctors, physical therapists, speech therapists and occupational therapists – to learn more. I quickly realized the information I was getting would be extremely valuable for other people with ALS and their loved ones.

This book has been a labor of love, one born of necessity and certainly one that aims to help those with ALS, their families, and their friends. All of the information in the book has been fact-checked by a medical professional for accuracy.

Introduction

a. What is ALS/Lou Gehrig's Disease?

Amyotrophic Lateral Sclerosis, one of the most common neuromuscular diseases in the world, attacks the nerves cells in the brain and in the spinal cord that control voluntary muscle movement. The motor neurons run from "the brain to the spinal cord and from the spinal cord to the muscles throughout the body," according to The ALS Association.

ALS causes the motor neurons to degenerate and to eventually die. The death of motor neurons results in the brain losing its ability to control the body's voluntary muscle movement, which often leads to total paralysis in the later stages of the disease. Due to the fact that the muscles cannot move, they begin to atrophy or waste away. When a muscle atrophies, it becomes smaller. You may notice that your loved one's arms, for example, look smaller than normal as the ALS progresses. That is because their muscles are atrophying and becoming smaller.

Those who suffer from ALS will find that, in the beginning, everyday movements, such as picking objects up and tying one's shoes, become more difficult. These symptoms are the result of the degeneration of the motor neurons. As the disease progresses, individuals with ALS have difficulty swallowing and often lose the ability to speak, requiring a speech generating device for communication. As the disease progresses and motor neurons begin to die, some ALS sufferers will suffer from complete paralysis.

ALS affects the nerves in the body that control voluntary movement and muscles. You may find it is more difficult to walk up the stairs or to pick up a child in the early stages of the disease because both of those actions are controlled by voluntary muscles in the arms and in the legs. Organs of the body that are involuntary, such as the beating of the heart and the digestive system, are not affected by ALS. As a result, the heart and digestive system generally continue to work normally, even with a diagnosis of ALS. Breathing, however, may be affected because, as the ALS Association notes, humans can hold their breath, which makes breathing, at least in part, a voluntary action.

ALS generally progresses very rapidly, claiming the lives of many patients within two to five years of their diagnosis. While ALS is classified as a terminal disease, life expectancy depends on the individual. Some people diagnosed with ALS, such as Stephen Hawking, have lived many years beyond the diagnosis, giving hope to those newly diagnosed with the motor neuron disease.

Progression of the disease depends on the individual. Many ALS patients are prescribed the medication Rilutek to help combat the affects of ALS while a variety of therapies can help make everyday life easier. Physical therapy in the early part of the disease allows individuals to keep muscles exercised, while occupational therapy will help you learn how to adapt your home and your life – such as installing bath rails and using assistive devices to help with eating and talking – to make coping with the affects of ALS easier.

Throughout this book, you will learn more about ALS – the symptoms, the testing you can expect as you work toward a diagnosis, how the disease generally progresses, common therapies, and assistive devices to make life easier, especially as the ALS progresses.

Furthermore, we will also delve into the financial considerations of being handed such a diagnosis and how caregivers can help their loved one, while also taking care of themselves.

b. Facts about ALS

A diagnosis of ALS is life changing for everyone involved – the person diagnosed with Lou Gehrig's Disease must come to terms with his disease and face his own mortality, while family and friends must deal with the life changes that will result as the ALS progresses and their loved one nears the end of life. Knowing what to expect from the disease, knowing what tools and coping mechanisms are available to make life easier, and knowing how to care for yourself if you are caring for a loved one with Lou Gehrig's Disease can make the journey much smoother.

Amyotrophic Lateral Sclerosis (ALS), most commonly referred to as Lou Gehrig's Disease, can strike anyone at any time of his or her life; it does not discriminate and those who suffer from the disease hail from every socioeconomic background, every race, and every country around the world. But, despite it being non-discriminatory, those who have been diagnosed with Lou Gehrig's Disease do share some common characteristics.

Approximately 93 percent of those who have been diagnosed with ALS are white and 60 percent are male. While more men than women typically are diagnosed with ALS in their 50s, that number tends to drop as men and women age. Men and women in their 60s and beyond generally have an equal likelihood of an ALS diagnosis.

It is important to remember that ALS can strike anyone at any age, but the most common timeframe for diagnosis is between the ages of 40 and 60, with the majority of ALS patients receiving a diagnosis in their 50s.

A notoriously difficult disease to diagnosis, which generally requires ruling out other diseases and illnesses that mimic it, Lou Gehrig's Disease is, first and foremost, not contagious and it is not an instant death sentence, although there is no cure. Half of ALS patients survive a minimum of three years following their diagnosis. Twenty percent of those diagnosed with ALS will live five or more years while 10 percent live 10 years or longer.

Research has found, according to The ALS Association, that overweight individuals and individuals who were at a normal weight at the time of diagnosis handle the affects of the disease better. Underweight individuals, or those who lose weight quickly after being diagnosed with ALS, do not fare as well in dealing with the symptoms of Lou Gehrig's Disease.

The ALS Association asserts that those diagnosed with ALS typically have a life expectancy of between three and five years. However, many people with ALS have beaten the odds and have lived even longer. Stephen Hawking, the famous British scientist, was diagnosed with ALS when he was only 21 years old. Doctors told him he would never see his 25th birthday.

Today, Hawking is 71 years old and has defied the odds, surviving a grim diagnosis and continuing with a brilliant career as a physicist, educator, author, and lecturer for more than five decades. (You can learn more about Hawking, including his battle with ALS, at his official website: http://www.hawking.org.uk/.)

c. Worldwide Statistics

Not as commonly known to the general public as cancer or other life-threatening diseases, ALS ranks as one of the most common neuromuscular diseases in the world, according to the National Institute of Neurological Disorders and Stroke. In fact, the University of California at San Diego's Center for ALS Research and Therapy has found that an individual is five times more likely to be diagnosed with Lou Gehrig's Disease than with Huntington's Disease while that same individual has an equal chance of developing ALS or multiple sclerosis.

Amyotrophic Lateral Sclerosis affects people, as we already mentioned, worldwide regardless of race, income, or where they live. Every year, an estimated 5,600 Americans are told they have Lou Gehrig's Disease. Nearly 1,100 people in the United Kingdom are diagnosed with Lou Gehrig's Disease every year, while three people who suffer from ALS die daily in the United Kingdom. Statistics show that 5 out of every 100,000 people, who are 20 years of age or older, die from complications of ALS every year in the United States.

5 percent of individuals are diagnosed with a familial or a genetic form of ALS, while 95 percent suffer from the sporadic form of Lou Gehrig's Disease. We will discuss the different types of Lou Gehrig's Disease (genetic, familial, and Guamanian in Chapter One).

d. ALS Strikes a Storied Baseball Player

The New York Yankees arguably have one of Major League Baseball's richest and most well-known histories. Say that to a Boston Red Sox fan, however, and you are likely to stir up a heated debate and some bitter feelings. It was the Yankees who bought perhaps baseball's most famous player, Babe Ruth, just as he was on the verge of athletic stardom, from the Red Sox. Ruth's departure from the Red Sox in 1919 to the Yankees simultaneously started the Red Sox on an 86 year drought without a pennant and put the Yankees on the road to one World Series Championship after another and to worldwide fame.

Many people, no matter where in the world you go, can identify the intertwined N and Y on the front of a dark navy baseball cap or on the front of a blue pinstriped jersey, or can name one of the game's most famous players – Babe Ruth, Lou Gehrig, Joe DiMaggio, Mickey Mantle, Roger Maris, and Yogi Berra are only a handful who have helped build the New York Yankee legend. Yankees' gear is worn by actors in Hollywood films and, perhaps most famously, George Costanza worked for the storied team on the popular American sitcom "Seinfeld" in the 1990s. The Yankees have, in a very real sense, become as synonymous with the American culture as apple pie.

It was back when Ruth first came to the Yankees, during the heyday of baseball in the early 20th century, when the game was still only about the game (and not the high salaries that often dominate today's baseball headlines), that the Yankees grabbed a hold of history both on and off the field due, in large part, to Ruth and, several years later, to a modest and talented first baseman named Lou Gehrig.

Gehrig, who earned the title of the Iron Horse of baseball during his 17 year career with the Yankees, was a hometown boy, born and raised in New York City, and a graduate of Columbia University. He left fans in awe over his hitting ability, one time knocking four homeruns out of the park in a single game, and his consecutive games played streak, which spanned 2,130 games, stood the test of time, until the Baltimore Orioles' Cal Ripken Jr. broke the record decades later in 1995. Gehrig's streak is even more impressive considering he was knocked unconscious by pitches in two games, yet managed to regain consciousness and continue playing in both of those games to maintain his streak.

Nothing, it seemed, could stop Gehrig, not even being rendered unconscious. But, during the 1939 season, the then-38-year-old Gehrig began to notice changes in his body. He was tired and could no longer move quite as fast or as well as he had earlier in the season. He was starting to have difficulty doing every day things like tying his shoes, signaling that something besides age was probably affecting his body.

Then, on May 2, 1939, after playing in every game of the season for the past 14 years, Gehrig instructed his manager, Joe McCarthy, to scratch him from the starting lineup.

The streak was over and, as Gehrig began a battle for his life, so was his Hall of Fame career in baseball. He left the game behind after tallying an impressive career that, to this day, is still talked about by broadcasters and fans. His career stats included an astonishing 2,130 consecutive games played over a 14 year period, a career batting average of .340, 493 homeruns, and 13 back-to-back seasons in which he tallied 100 RBIs (Runs Batted In). He also earned six World Series titles during his career with the Yankees.

Gehrig sought help from the Mayo Clinic, where he was diagnosed with Amyotrophic Lateral Sclerosis (ALS). Following his official diagnosis, Gehrig made his final appearance, fully dressed in his Yankees' uniform, at the Yankee Stadium on July 4, 1939.

On that day, he delivered what many in baseball consider one of the game's most inspiring speeches, particularly in light of the disease with which he had been diagnosed. In his speech, he illustrated the same grace with which he had played the American pastime of baseball, telling the world and future generations:

"Fans, for the past two weeks you have been reading about the bad break I got. Yet today I consider myself the luckiest man on the face of this earth. I have been in ballparks for seventeen years and have never received anything but kindness and encouragement from you fans.

When the New York Giants, a team you would give your right arm to beat, and vice versa, sends you a gift - that's something. When everybody down to the groundskeepers and those boys in white coats remember you with trophies - that's something. When you have a wonderful mother-in-law who takes sides with you in squabbles with her own daughter - that's something. When you have a father and a mother who work all their lives so you can have an education and build your body - it's a blessing. When you have a wife who has been a tower of strength and shown more courage than you dreamed existed - that's the finest I know.

So I close in saying that I may have had a tough break, but I have an awful lot to live for."

Gehrig's speech, in which he also praised the famous players and managers with whom he played the game for 17 seasons, is routinely played on scoreboards in baseball stadiums across America and Gary Cooper played the Iron Horse in the Hollywood film "The Pride of the Yankees," which shared Gehrig's tale, in 1942. But, Gehrig would not be there to see that portrayal.

The Iron Horse of baseball succumbed to ALS on June 2, 1941, dying in his sleep less than two years after his diagnosis. But, with his diagnosis and subsequent death, Lou Gehrig's name became synonymous with the disease that ended his career and his life. In a very real sense, Lou Gehrig put a face to ALS, a disease that many had arguably never heard of, unless directly affected, until Lou Gehrig, baseball's Iron Horse, made headlines with his diagnosis.

Today, when the media features a story on Amyotrophic Lateral Sclerosis, it typically mentions that ALS is "also known as Lou Gehrig's Disease, after the famous New York Yankee."

Chapter One: Types of ALS

a. Sporadic ALS

Sporadic ALS is the most common type of amyotrophic lateral sclerosis, the cause of between 90 and 95 percent of all cases of ALS in the world. While researchers have yet to pinpoint an exact cause of Lou Gehrig's Disease, experts point to several possible different causes of ALS, including:

Possible Causes of Sporadic ALS

Free radicals
Molecules with unpaired electrons are called free radicals, which we all have in our bodies. Generally, however, our bodies are able to neutralize the free radicals and prevent them from overproducing. Some individuals with ALS, however, have been found to have an abundance of free radicals, which become toxic. Those toxins then damage cells, which could result in the appearance of ALS.

Abnormalities in the immune system
Individuals with ALS have been found to have abnormal proteins that are created by the immune system, while others suffer from a greater number of immune disorders. Essentially, it is believed that the immune system attacks the nerve cells, which could lead to an increase of calcium in individual cells. The result may be the degeneration of motor neurons.

Midochondrial defects

Mitochondria, which is extremely susceptible to oxidative damage, produces free radicals. The mitochondria may be damaged by the free radicals, which results in a degeneration of nerve cells.

Toxins

While there is no conclusive evidence that toxins are a contributing factor to Lou Gehrig's Disease, researchers continue to look at the role that certain toxins – such as radiation, solvents, and heavy metals – play in the development of ALS in some individuals.

Chemical Imbalance

ALS patients have been found to possess an abundance of glutamate in their bodies, which according to the Mayo Clinic, is "a chemical messenger in the brain, around the nerve cells in their spinal fluid. Too much glutamate is known to be toxic to some nerve cells."

b. Genetic or Familial ALS

Lou Gehrig's Disease can be inherited, although the likelihood of hereditary ALS is typically very small at between five and 10 percent. Doctors generally distinguish between a familial case of ALS and a sporadic case of ALS by discussing the individual's family history. Have there been family members that have been diagnosed with ALS? If the answer is yes, the ALS is likely genetic.

Sometimes, however, it is not that easy. An individual may have been adopted, so knowing family history may be difficult or even impossible. If an individual has a family member who passed away at an early age but does not know why, doctors will generally want to know at what age that family member passed away and whether that family member had problems with walking and speech that got progressively worse with time, which could give clues as to whether the death could have been the result of Lou Gehrig's Disease.

Remember, however, that familial ALS is relatively rare compared to incidents of sporadic ALS.

c. Genetic testing: Are your children likely to develop ALS?

If a family member has genetic ALS, will his or her children or grandchildren develop Lou Gehrig's Disease later in their lives? If your father or mother has ALS, will you, too, be diagnosed with it at some point in your life? Will your children be at risk for developing ALS? Such questions often lead those with a family history of ALS to seek out genetic testing.

Testing is often done on family members who have a loved one with ALS, who have a loved one who is showing symptoms of ALS, or who have a family history of ALS. Genetic testing may also be appropriate for people who have been adopted or those individuals who do not know their family history. If an individual's parent died at an early age, and the child does not know why, genetic testing may be recommended.

While genetic testing is available, it is not conclusive and it does not mean that a person will develop ALS. Alternately, even if the genetic testing offers a negative result, you could still develop ALS. Only certain genes that cause familial ALS have been found.

In other words:

A positive result = genetic cause of familial ALS has been found

A negative result = no genetic cause of familial ALS has been found

If you have family members with Lou Gehrig's Disease and want genetic testing, you will find it is a generally simple, though often long, process. You will have a blood test done, which will then be sent to a laboratory for analysis. The lab technician will extract your DNA from the blood and will test it using a single strand or by using sequencing.

The time frame and the cost for genetic testing can vary greatly depending on the laboratory with which you are working. However, as a general rule, genetic testing generally takes between two and three months to complete. Costs for the testing can range anywhere from a few hundred dollars to a few thousand dollars.

If you are not experiencing any symptoms commonly associated with ALS and you are not sure whether or not to get tested for familial ALS, discuss the possibility with your doctor. Some people prefer not to know whether they possess the gene that could potentially result in them or their children developing ALS, because that worry would be too great for them. Others prefer to know, which allows them to keep a close eye on research as researchers work for a cure for ALS. Whether or not to get tested when you are not showing symptoms is a highly personal decision. You may decide to get tested while your sibling may not.

Keep in mind that genetic testing is not the same as a diagnosis of ALS. If you are showing symptoms, such as muscle weakness, generally associated with Lou Gehrig's Disease, you should schedule an appointment with your doctor. We will discuss how ALS is diagnosed in Chapter Four, but briefly, you will undergo numerous tests to rule out other illnesses and diseases that mirror ALS before you can be definitively diagnosed with Lou Gehrig's Disease.

d. Guamanian ALS

Most literature on ALS touches on the Guamanian form of Amyotrophic Lateral Sclerosis, but it does not seem to be as prevalent today. Native Guamanians, living in Guam, and the Trust Territories of the Pacific between 1940 and 1965, were diagnosed with ALS at a startlingly high rate. During that time period, ALS was the leading cause of death for native Guamanians and an estimated 400 natives out of 100,000 received a diagnosis of ALS. Today, that number has dropped dramatically to 22 incidents for every 100,000 natives.

Researchers believe that the high rate of ALS during that 25 year time period could have been the result of the natives' diet. At the time, Guamanians consumed a high level of fruit bats in their diet. Fruit bats eat nuts, which are poisonous, from the cycad tree.

While no clear connection has yet been formed between the Guamanians' diet and the high incidence of ALS, the rate of ASL diagnoses dropped drastically after the fruit bat became extinct in Guam and the Guamanians began importing bats from Samoa. Those bats did not feed on cycad trees.

Chapter Two: Warning Signs, Common Symptoms of ALS

Despite it being one of the most common neuromuscular diseases in the world, Lou Gehrig's Disease is still notoriously difficult to diagnose because it mirrors symptoms of other diseases, such as multiple sclerosis. Added to that difficulty in securing a diagnosis is the fact that many people have symptoms that are so small in the beginning that they do not even realize something is wrong until the disease begins to progress and the muscle weakness becomes progressively worse.

In addition to ALS mimicking other diseases, those who are eventually diagnosed with Lou Gehrig's Disease have varying symptoms in the beginning. Everyone experiences symptoms differently. However, there are some common warning signs of which you should be aware.

a. General Muscle Weakness

One of the first symptoms of Lou Gehrig's Disease for many with ALS is a general weakness in the arms, legs, or hands. Often, the weakness is so small at first, that many people simply dismiss the weakness as fatigue. You may begin to notice that you have trouble walking or climbing the stairs. Even stepping up onto a curb may require extra effort. You may have trouble holding a pen or picking up a brush and brushing your hair. Lou Gehrig, before he was diagnosed, began having difficulty tying his shoes.

If you notice such weakness, consult with your doctor, especially if you notice it becoming progressively worse. An estimated 60 percent of those with ALS experience some form of muscle weakness, according to the ALS Association.

Other incidents of general muscle weakness may include:

- Difficulty in lifting your foot (it may drop on its own when you try to lift it onto a curb, for example)

- Tripping over small things, such as a piece of carpet

- A general clumsiness (which may be ignored if you are typically clumsy already)

- Cramps, predominately in the legs, hands, and feet

- Difficulty chewing food

Muscle weakness, in the beginning, may be predominant in one area of the body, such as the hand, or on one side of the body.

b. Difficulty Swallowing or Breathing

ALS attacks the motor neurons that control voluntary muscles, which often affect swallowing and breathing, especially as the disease progresses. Like with muscle weakness, people often misplace the difficulty breathing or shortness of breath as simply exerting themselves too much. Breathing problems become significantly worse as the disease progresses.

c. Muscle Spasms

If you have ever experienced a muscle spasm, especially for the first time, you know how uncomfortable and downright painful it can be. In the early onset of ALS, muscle spasms may present themselves in the form of tiny twitches. You may be sitting down, for example, and your arm or leg begins to twitch. Such twitches or muscle spasms, especially in conjunction with other symptoms, may be a warning sign of ALS.

d. Trouble Speaking

We all trip over our words sometimes, which may be why some people dismiss any problems they initially have with their speech. Early warning signs of ALS include slurring of your speech and having difficulty, where you previously did not, pronouncing your words. You may also find that you have a difficult time speaking as loudly as you would like.

e. Areas Not Affected

Lou Gehrig's Disease only affects voluntary muscles. Those with ALS generally maintain their five senses, including smell, taste, touch, hearing, and sight. Most people do not have to worry about problems with the heart, the bladder, or the eyes.

As Stephen Hawking has proven over the past five decades, people can and do live productive lives even with a diagnosis of ALS. Individuals with ALS, even if they lose their ability to speak, can use speech generating devices to make communication possible and can continue breathing with the assistance of an invasive ventilator.

f. Keep Track of Your Symptoms

Maybe you have just started noticing that you are having a little more difficulty doing everyday things. You trip over small things or even over nothing at all. You get tired when you try to brush your hair; the brush just feels so much heavier these days. You have difficulty swallowing sometimes, even when you are eating soup or drinking tea. You have trouble holding a pen and writing or you notice that your legs seem to be a lot weaker than they were just a few days ago.

Start keeping track of your symptoms in a symptom diary. Write down what you are experiencing and when you experience it. As tedious as it may sound, be sure to write down every incident, no matter how small you think it is. You may not think the fact that you felt a little twitching in your foot yesterday is a big deal, but that small twitch could be a big clue for your doctor or neurologist. When you make that first appointment with your doctor, take your symptom diary with you. Showing your doctor your symptoms that way could help him have an easier time ruling out other diseases or illnesses which commonly mirror ALS and could help you get the right diagnosis faster.

g. Make an Appointment with Your Doctor

If you notice any of the symptoms commonly associated with ALS, make an appointment with your doctor to determine if testing should be done. As we already mentioned, ALS is difficult to diagnose. In Chapter Four, we will discuss the diseases and illnesses that ALS mirrors, the tests that are generally done to reach a definitive diagnosis of ALS, and how to cope with the emotional and practical aspects of dealing with an ALS diagnosis. We will discuss what to expect when the ALS progresses in Chapter Five.

The sooner you see a doctor after experiencing such symptoms, the easier it will be to get a correct diagnosis. It can often take more than nine months to get a correct diagnosis of ALS due to several factors. First, most people simply brush off their symptoms, attributing it to fatigue or some other reason, and may wait as long as six months before they make an appointment with the doctor.

Second, a doctor may not refer the individual to a neurologist because he does not suspect Lou Gehrig's Disease. As a result, the disease continues to progress undiagnosed and the individual may not be referred to a neurologist for as long as seven months from that first doctor's appointment.

Third, even if an individual does go to a neurologist, the neurologist may not initially suspect ALS. Sometimes individuals, who are eventually diagnosed with ALS, do not originally display common symptoms. The individual's symptoms may not be rapidly progressing, or the individual's symptoms do not yet meet the general criteria for being diagnosed with ALS, so the neurologist may offer another diagnosis. That diagnosis will eventually be ruled out for the correct diagnosis of ALS. The time between the wrong diagnosis and the ALS diagnosis could be months.

To ensure you get the ball rolling on a correct diagnosis early, make an appointment with your doctor if you experience any symptoms associated with ALS. It is better to start now than to wait, especially if you do have ALS, so you can start medication and therapy as soon as possible.

Chapter Three: Diagnosing ALS

a. How ALS is Diagnosed

You have begun experiencing symptoms that are common with Lou Gehrig's Disease and you have made an appointment with your family physician to find out just what is going on and if you really do have ALS. What can you expect from that first doctor's appointment?

Before you start what can amount to a thorough and a lengthy testing process, you will first just meet with your doctor. Your doctor will talk with you about your medical history, asking you pertinent questions such as: Has anyone in your family been diagnosed with ALS? Has anyone in your family died at an early age, but you did not know the cause of death? Has anyone in your family suffered from a progression of muscle weakness?

Once you have gone over your medical history with your doctor, he will probably go through a series of tests in the office to see how well certain functions – balance, coordination, smell, sight, reflex, and muscle tone – are working.

Your doctor may be able to eliminate some diseases based on the results of the tests he performs and he may recommend that you see a neurologist for additional testing.

b. Diseases/Illnesses that Mirror ALS

One of the biggest challenges doctors face in offering the correct diagnosis of ALS is the fact that it mirrors numerous other diseases and illnesses, including muscular dystrophy, stroke, and multiple sclerosis. Your doctor will first require that you go through a series of tests, which we will discuss in the next section, to rule out other diseases or illnesses that may be causing your symptoms.

Muscular Dystrophy

While there are several different types of Muscular Dystrophy, several of the symptoms of each are common with ALS, according to the Mayo Clinic, including:

- Progressive muscle weakness
- Tripping easily and frequently
- Difficulty swallowing

To learn more about Muscular Dystrophy, visit the Muscular Dystrophy Association at http://mda.org/.

Multiple Sclerosis

Like Lou Gehrig's Disease, Multiple Sclerosis is a life-threatening disease that drastically alters a patient's lifestyle and quality of life. The National Multiple Sclerosis Society provides a long list of common and less common symptoms of those with MS, many of which mirror the symptoms of ALS, including:

- Trouble walking
- Difficulty with coordination and balance
- Fatigue
- Problems swallowing
- Breathing problems
- Problems with speaking
- Emotional changes

To learn more about Multiple Sclerosis, visit the National Multiple Sclerosis Society at http://www.nationalmssociety.org/about-multiple-sclerosis/what-we-know-about-ms/symptoms/index.aspx.

Stroke

Some ALS patients may, at first, confuse their ALS symptoms, thinking that they actually had a stroke. The symptoms of a stroke are strikingly similar to the symptoms of ALS, including the following, which all occur suddenly, according to The National Stroke Association:

- Loss of balance
- Loss of coordination
- Muscle weakness in the face, arms, or legs
- Difficulty speaking
- Difficulty walking

To learn more about strokes and how to prevent strokes, visit The National Stroke Association at http://www.stroke.org/sitePageServer?pagename=symp.

These are just a few of the many illnesses and diseases that mimic ALS. You can now see why an ALS diagnosis is not so easy. And, because there is not a test to definitively diagnose Lou Gehrig's Disease, your doctor will insist on ruling out other possible causes of your symptoms.

c. Tests to Diagnose ALS

In an effort to correctly diagnosis a patient with ALS, doctors may require that individuals go through a battery of other tests, which will help rule out other illnesses and diseases that often mimic Lou Gehrig's Disease.

MRI

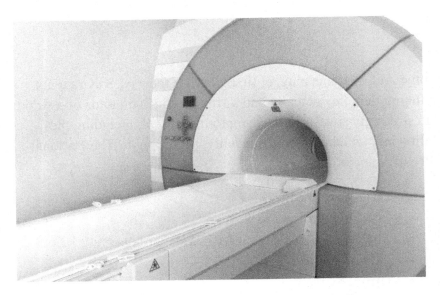

An MRI – or Magnetic Resonance Imaging – will allow your neurologist to get a clear view of your nervous system. MRIs use magnets and radio waves to give physicians a detailed look at different parts of the body. You may be required to have an MRI done on your spine or on your brain, which will help your doctor rule out other illnesses or diseases similar to ALS.

Blood/Urine

You have probably already had dozens of blood and urine tests in your lifetime. A blood or urine test, which you can generally have done right at your doctor's office, will help rule out other diseases or illnesses. Your blood may also be tested to determine the hormone levels of your thyroid and parathyroid, according to the ALS Association, and your urine may be tested for heavy metals.

If you have a history of Lou Gehrig's Disease in your family, your doctor may also have the blood tested for familial ALS. Refer to Chapter One, in which we discussed genetic testing for familial ALS.

Electromyogram

ALS affects the motor neurons that control voluntary muscle movement, leaving the sensory nerves intact. That means that people with ALS generally maintain their normal sense of hearing, sight, smell, sound, and touch. An electromyogram, or EMG, will test to see if your motor neurons are functioning properly. An EMG will require you to have tiny electrodes inserted into your muscles which will then test if and how well your motor neurons are functioning. If they are not functioning but your sensory nerves are working as they should be, you are exhibiting a classic symptom of ALS.

Respiratory Tests

Your doctor may require you to undergo respiratory testing. Respiratory testing will allow the doctor to see if you have a problem with the muscles that allow you to breathe.

Nerve Conduction

Nerve conduction will help assess how well and whether your muscles and nerves are working. You will have two electrodes placed on your skin. The nurse will then turn on the electrodes. You may feel a small shock as the electrodes move through the nerves. The shock will measure how well the electrical impulses in the nerve signals are functioning.

Muscle Biopsy

A muscle biopsy is a simple procedure that requires a nurse to take a small amount of muscle tissue from you, which will then be tested for such problems as Muscular Dystrophy or Myositis.

Spinal Tap

During a spinal tap, a small needle will be inserted in your lower back to retrieve spinal fluid, which will then be tested for abnormal cells. Spinal taps, however, are generally not done except in rare occasions when the individual exhibits abnormality in the spinal nerves.

By the time you complete whatever tests the doctor has ordered for you, your doctor should have a fairly good idea of which disease, and if it is ALS, you are facing. However, before you can receive an official diagnosis of Lou Gehrig's Disease, you must first meet certain criteria.

d. Necessary Criteria for an ALS Diagnosis

To be definitively diagnosed with Lou Gehrig's Disease, individuals must first meet specific criteria called the El Escorial Criteria for the Diagnosis of Amyotrophic Lateral Sclerosis (ALS). That criteria requires:

- Individuals must be experiencing symptoms that are progressing and moving toward other parts of the body or that have spread within a region of the body.

- A clinical examination that finds that upper motor neurons have started degenerating. The upper motor neurons are found in the brain.

- A clinical examination or specialized testing that finds the lower motor neurons have started degenerating. The lower motor neurons can be found in the brainstem and the spinal cord.

- Ruling out other diseases as the cause of symptoms; a lack of evidence that another disease or illness may be causing the individual's symptoms.

Once those criteria have been met, an individual will be given an official diagnosis of Amyotrophic Lateral Sclerosis.

e. Should You Get a Second Opinion?

Many people who are diagnosed with a life-altering, terminal illness opt to get a second opinion, no matter how good the reputation of their first doctor. If you are not sure whether the diagnosis of ALS is correct or you just want peace of mind to know that the diagnosis is correct, consider getting a second opinion.

Statistics illustrate the validity of a second opinion. Approximately 15 percent of people diagnosed with ALS later learn that they, in fact, do not have Lou Gehrig's Disease.

Alternately, an estimated 40 percent of those who are eventually diagnosed with ALS are first told they have another disease, according to the ALS Association.

Do not worry about offending your current doctor because you want a second opinion. Doctors are professionals and understand that patients sometimes need additional confirmation, especially when facing a terminal diagnosis. Inform your doctor you want a second opinion. He may be able to refer you to a neurologist who specializes in or who has experience with ALS.

Do not just go to any neurologist. It is essential you find a doctor with experience with ALS. Some neurologists specialize in neuromuscular diseases, and that is the type of doctor you want. To find neurologists with experience in ALS, consider contacting:

- The American Academy of Neurology: 1-800-879-1960

- The ALS Association's Referral Line: 1-800-782-4747

You may also be able to find referrals by contacting hospitals and neurology specialists in your area. Make sure you ask questions about any neurologist you decide to see to determine his or her experience with ALS and knowledge of the disease.

A second opinion, depending on your insurance, may require you to pay out-of-pocket expenses. If you are in the United States and are currently covered by Medicare, you can contact Medicare to determine if a second opinion would be covered. (You can reach Medicare in the United States at 1-800-MEDICARE or 1-800-633-4227.)

If you have insurance, be sure to call your insurance company before you go for your second opinion. That way, you know if it is covered or if you have to meet certain criteria to have the visit covered.

f. Coping With a Diagnosis of ALS

You or a loved one has just been diagnosed with Lou Gehrig's Disease. Maybe it is the first time you have really heard of ALS and you are overwhelmed because you just do not know what to expect. Maybe you have heard of ALS before and are in shock over the diagnosis.

Being diagnosed with ALS is not easy on anyone: the person who has just been diagnosed must now face his or her own mortality and the family and friends must now deal with the fact that their loved one has been diagnosed with a disease that will eventually take his or her life.

How do you cope with a life-changing diagnosis like Lou Gehrig's Disease? Everyone deals with life-altering news differently, but in this section we are going to discuss some ways that may help you to deal with the emotional aspects of a terminal diagnosis and the practical steps you are now going to have to consider as you move forward and begin dealing with the everyday consequences of ALS.

The Emotional Aspects of an ALS Diagnosis

You are likely experiencing a mix of emotions after hearing the ALS diagnosis. Learning how to deal with the emotional aspects of ALS can be just as important to your overall mental and physical health as learning how to make adjustments in your life for the changes that will come as the ALS progresses.

Give yourself time to accept the diagnosis. Whether you are the one who has received the ALS diagnosis or your loved one has been diagnosed with ALS, you have just been hit with something that is going to change your life forever from this point on. You may experience a range of emotions and you may go through the steps of grief. That is okay. It is normal to grieve for what you have lost and for what you will lose with an ALS diagnosis.

Allow yourself to feel whatever you feel. If you are angry, that is okay. If you are sad, that is okay. If you are frustrated, that is okay. Give yourself the time to deal with your emotions and to accept the diagnosis. It may take you longer than another loved one or vice versa. There is no right way to deal with a terminal illness.

Join a support group. Whether you have been diagnosed with ALS or a loved one has been diagnosed with ALS, you are now part of a community that understands and knows what you are going through. Others can sympathize and empathize and be there for you as best as they can.

Only someone in your situation truly understands what you are going through. A support group can help you cope with life's changes as a result of ALS. You will make friends and have people, who are in the same situation you are in, to whom you can turn when you need to vent or to cry. They may also offer advice, and vice versa, on how to deal with different situations and for treatments that may help.

Support groups exist for both those who have been diagnosed with ALS and for loved ones and caregivers of someone with ALS. Check out the ALS Association or the Muscular Dystrophy Association for support groups in your area. You may also want to talk with your doctor, who can tell you about any local support groups. Many hospitals and medical facilities also keep lists of support groups.

Share your feelings with loved ones and vice versa. You and your loved ones are all going through an emotional time and you are all likely to deal with a roller coaster of emotions. Share your feelings with your loved ones and encourage them to do the same with you.

Have hope. Sometimes a positive attitude can have more of an impact on your health than you realize. The doctor may have told you that many ALS patients only live three to five years, but many also survive much longer. Ten percent live more than five years while another 10 percent live longer than 10 years. An ALS diagnosis is not an instant death sentence. Researchers are constantly working toward new advances, treatments, and a cure for ALS. It may happen in your lifetime. Do not give up hope. (We will discuss advances in research in Chapter Fourteen.)

Remember, you have not changed. You may have just been handed a diagnosis of ALS, but you are the same person you were before your doctor ever uttered the term "ALS." You still have an identity and a life that you have built before ALS. Your body will go through changes as your disease progresses, but you are not your disease. ALS does not define you.

Surround yourself with positive people. You are dealing with something that not everyone can understand. You are likely to go through periods of depression and have negative thoughts. You do not need other people to do that for you. Spend time with friends and loved ones who will lift you up and remind you of the positives in life and avoid those who bring too much negativity with them.

Consider counseling. Many times, those with ALS and their loved ones need help processing their feelings and dealing with what is going on and what is to come. Counseling can be a life preserver. Many hospitals have social workers who can connect you or your loved ones with counselors. But, counselors come in many forms, and may be a psychologist; a pastor, a priest, a rabbi, or another religious figure; a psychiatrist, or even a good friend.

g. The Practical Aspects

Dealing with the emotional aspects of ALS is just as important as dealing with the practical parts of your diagnosis. Again, whether you have been diagnosed with ALS or you will be caring for a loved one who has been diagnosed with ALS, you must start making decisions.

Start treatment as soon as possible. Most ALS patients take Rilutek for their ALS, which we will discuss in Chapter Six, and begin physical therapy and occupational therapy. Getting started with treatment could slow the progression of the ALS and it may make its progression easier on you.

Be in charge of your treatment. You will have plenty of people, from doctors to family and friends, supporting you and advising you. In the end, your course of treatment and how you live and choose to die is up to only one person: You. Take charge of your treatment and make the decisions you want.

Plan ahead. You may survive your diagnosis for the next 20 or 30 years. But, there will come a time that you are no longer able to care for yourself. Who will care for you? If you cannot make medical decisions yourself, who will make those decisions for you? What type of end of life care do you want? Will you stay at home for your final days? Will you have a nurse come in if your caregiver can no longer provide for all of your needs? Or, do you prefer moving to an assisted living facility in the final stages of your life, to have the around the clock care you may need?

What do you want after your death? Some people donate their tissue, which we will talk about in Chapter Twelve, to research while others donate their bodies to help researchers work toward a cure for ALS.

All of these are very difficult subjects about which you will have to think and to make decisions, so you can remain in charge of your care throughout the rest of your life and into your end of life.

Create a living will. A living will stipulates what you want done in case you slip into a vegetative state or into a coma from which you may never wake. Tubes can keep the human body alive for many years. Do you want tubes to keep you alive if you slip into a vegetative state or a coma? Or, do you want to be removed from lifesaving devices in such a situation? A living will stipulates exactly what you want. You may want something completely different than your spouse or children. Your spouse or children may not want to let you go in such a situation and, without a living will, may keep you alive, even if that is not what you wanted, just because they do not want to lose you.

You have the final say with a living will, but it is important to make sure you tell others your wishes and designate someone, who knows and will respect what you want, to make important decisions for you when you cannot do it yourself.

Prepare your home. Your body is going to go through a lot of changes as your ALS progresses. As a result, you are going to need to accommodate your home to prepare for those changes. We will discuss how to prepare your home and assistive devices that can make living with ALS easier in detail in Chapter Eight. But, briefly, you can tailor your home to the changes that your body will go through by adding bath rails in the tub and ramps throughout the inside and outside of your home. You will also want to be fitted for a wheelchair early in your disease and well before you need it as it generally takes time to order and have a wheelchair custom made.

Now that you have an ALS diagnosis, you have a lot to think about and a lot to do. But, before you do anything, remember to allow yourself the opportunity to go through the emotions you are feeling and to come to terms with your diagnosis. Be kind to yourself as you embark on this new journey in your life and remain hopeful. Researchers are working hard to find a cure and to find ways to slow the progress of ALS down.

Chapter Four: What to Expect As ALS Progresses

How fast Lou Gehrig's Disease progresses really depends on the individual. Everyone is different. No official classification of stages of Amyotrophic Lateral Sclerosis exists, although researchers have proposed a six stage classification system for ALS.

Those six stages, according to researchers cited in the Brain: A Journal of Neurology would include:

- The first stage, stage 1, signifies the onset of ALS symptoms in a patient's first region.
- The second stage, stage 2A, denotes the patient's diagnosis of ALS.
- In stage 2B, patients begin to experience symptoms of ALS in the second region of their bodies.
- In the third stage, patients begin to experience ALS symptoms in the third region.
- In the fourth stage, stage 4A, patients must have a gastrostomy.
- In the final stage, stage 4B, the patient requires non-invasive assistance with breathing.

Researchers continue to study ALS and the benefits of creating an official six stage classification system. However, because that information is not yet official, we are going to discuss the progression of ALS, using the Muscular Dystrophy Association's classification system. The Muscular Dystrophy Association segregates ALS into three distinct stages: the early stage, the middle stage, and the last stage.

Chapter Four: What to Expect as ALS Progresses

a. The First Stage of ALS

The early stages of Lou Gehrig's Disease may present symptoms that are so small you do not even recognize there is a problem. You may notice a variety of symptoms, which we touched on briefly in Chapter Two, including:

- Fatigue
- Muscle cramps
- Muscle twitches or spasms
- Slurred or distorted speech
- General muscle weakness of the hands, arms, legs, and those muscles required for breathing and for swallowing

Often, as we have already discussed, the symptoms are so slight that individuals simply ignore them until they start to become worse. During the early stage of ALS, your life probably won't change very much, and you may not even know that you have ALS.

b. The Middle Stage of ALS

The middle stage of ALS may start with you being diagnosed with Lou Gehrig's Disease. By the middle stage, your symptoms of ALS will become more noticeable and will begin spreading to other areas of your body. It is likely that you will no longer be able to drive and if you fall, you may no longer be able to lift yourself up. You will need more assistance from others during the middle stage to do such things as tying your shoes and buttoning your buttons.

The middle stage of ALS, according to the Muscular Dystrophy Association, often introduces a variety of new symptoms, such as:

- You may begin drooling as you have difficulty managing the excess saliva.

- You may start having trouble swallowing, which could result in difficulty eating and choking.

- You may start to experience breathing problems. For example, you may not be able to breathe properly while lying down, requiring you to use additional pillows or to sleep in a recliner. At this point, your doctor may recommend the non-invasive breathing assistance of a facial mask.

- You may deal with Involuntary Emotional Expression Disorder (IEED), or Pseudobulbar Affect (PBA). With IEED, you cannot control your emotions and may begin laughing or crying uncontrollably for no reason at all. You may, for example, feel perfectly content when you begin to suddenly cry for no reason.

c. The Late Stage of ALS

As you progress into the late stage of ALS, you are nearing the end of life. By this point in the disease, you will need assistance to care for you and may you be unable to do much on your own. In the late stage of ALS:

- You may lose your ability to speak, which can be rectified with a speech generating device.

- You may no longer be able to feed or drink by yourself and may require a feeding tube to ensure you get the proper nutrition. Often, swallowing becomes increasingly difficult and dangerous as the ALS progresses.

- Your breathing problems are likely to worsen, and you may consider using an invasive ventilator to do the breathing for you. A ventilator requires around the clock care from a trained professional or a caregiver who has been trained in how the ventilator works.

During the last stage, you and your caregiver may want to consider hospice care, which will help relieve some of your caregiver's responsibilities and provide you with a team of medical professionals (doctors, nurses, social workers, etc.) to help keep you comfortable. Hospice care typically takes place at home, although you may be admitted to a hospice house. Hospice care may also be available if you are in a nursing facility or in the hospital.

d. Common Health Problems with ALS

We already discussed the common symptoms in the early stages of ALS in Chapter Two. Now we will take a closer look at the different problems you may experience as your ALS progresses.

Constipation

Some people with ALS deal with constipation for a number of reasons. Constipation is often a side effect of the medications used to treat symptoms of ALS. In addition, when your activity level decreases as your ALS progresses, you may also deal with constipation. Many patients with ALS will drink less water and other liquids so they have to go to the bathroom less frequently and diet changes often occur because of swallowing issues. As a result, individuals with ALS do not get the fiber and proper nutrition they need, resulting in constipation.

Combating constipation is often fairly straightforward. Make sure you eat a proper diet. You may work with a dietician or your speech pathologist may provide suggestions on how to eat even when swallowing is difficult.

Fatigue

Fatigue is often an early symptom of ALS and will continue throughout the progression of the disease. With the assistance of your medical team, including a speech pathologist and occupational therapist, you will learn how to avoid fatigue by using assistive devices, such as a wheelchair, and by using different techniques to conserve energy. For example, early in the disease, you may want to obtain a handicap permit from your local DMV, so you are not tired just from walking from the parking space into the store or the doctor's office.

Frontotemporal Dementia (FTD)

Some people with ALS develop a form of dementia called frontotemporal dementia or FTD. Those ALS patients who develop FTD may exhibit symptoms such as antisocial behavior, personality changes, or difficulty identifying common objects. To date, there are no effective treatments for those suffering from FTD.

Difficulty Talking

Many individuals with ALS lose the ability to speak as the ALS progresses. Initially, you may experience slurred speech or trip over your words as you speak. However, working with a speech pathologist, which we will discuss in Chapter Seven, will allow you to learn how to communicate when your voice no longer works. Speech generating devices allow you to speak using your recorded voice or a computerized voice.

Drooling

A common problem for those with ALS is excessive saliva. In fact, you may not actually be making more saliva. You just may not be able to swallow all of the saliva you do make. During the early stages of ALS, you may be able to control the problem and avoid drooling by making a conscious effort to swallow more often.

As the ALS progresses, you may begin to experience difficulty swallowing, so drooling becomes a problem. Some people with ALS have found that, at least in the beginning when their muscles still allow, using a Kleenex or a cloth to wipe away excess drool is sufficient for controlling the problem. If that is not enough, some people opt to use a suction machine, which will remove the excess saliva from your mouth. You can even purchase a portable suction machine that runs on batteries, allowing you to take it with you wherever you go.

If you find that drooling is just too much of a problem for you, contact you doctor who can prescribe a medication to help. Medications used to control drooling include Robinul, Elavil, Pro-Banthine and Pamelor.

Your doctor will provide you with the exact dosage, instructions on how to take the medication (with or without food), and the potential side effects.

Involuntary Emotional Expression Disorder (IEED)

Involuntary Emotional Expression Disorder (IEED), or Pseudobulbar Affect (PBA), is a neurological disorder commonly associated with ALS. Essentially, the person with ALS has sudden and uncontrollable fits of laughter or crying. You may be laughing or crying uncontrollably, even though you do not feel happy or sad. You simply cannot control those emotions and do not know when the IEED will strike. IEED can be treated with medication, Nuedexta, prescribed by your doctor.

Respiratory Issues

As your muscles become weaker as your ALS progresses, you may start having breathing difficulties, which we will discuss further in Chapter Seven. You may not be able to breathe properly if you lie down flat and may only get restful sleep if you are sitting up. A non-invasive face mask can help you with breathing, or you may opt for an invasive approach of using a ventilator as breathing on your own becomes too difficult.

Many individuals with ALS also develop swallowing problems, as the muscles in their throat and mouths begin to weaken and atrophy. Swallowing problems could inadvertently cause respiratory issues. You may have difficulty swallowing, which causes you to choke or to cough, and you may aspirate food into your lungs. (Your doctor may recommend a feeding tube to help avoid aspiration.) That aspiration could lead to dangerous respiratory issues, such as pneumonia. Pneumonia is extremely dangerous and could and does result in the death of some patients with ALS.

Slurred speech

Slurred and nasal-sounding speech may begin in the early stages of ALS or may take a while to progress; it all depends on the individual. As we will discuss in Chapter Seven, many individuals with Lou Gehrig's Disease lose the ability to speak but can still communicate verbally with assistive devices and non-verbally using facial expressions and hand gestures. A speech pathologist can work with you to provide you with ways to conserve energy when speaking and can offer suggestions for assistive devices that will make communicating easier for you and for those to whom you are speaking.

e. End of Life

The most common cause of death in those with ALS is respiratory failure. Respiratory failure is generally a process that occurs over a period of several months, according to the Mayo Clinic, with that process typically beginning between three and five years from the time of diagnosis. Remember, however, that many people beat that initial three to five year lifespan and go on to live for 10, 15, and even 20 years or more.

Chapter Five: Treatment: Medication

a. Rilutek

The most commonly used medication to slow down the progression of Lou Gehrig's Disease is Rilutek. In fact, Rilutek is the only drug on the market today that has been approved for treatment of ALS by the Food and Drug Administration (FDA) in the United States. All other medications individuals with ALS are prescribed are generally in an attempt to help curb the effects of ALS, such as cramping, fatigue, pain, depression, and constipation.

Individuals with ALS have mixed results with Rilutek. The medication slows the progress of the ALS down in some people, while it does not have the same effect in others. However, many doctors prescribe Rilutek in an attempt to slow the progression of the disease.

Side effects

Rilutek affects different people in different ways. You may experience one, some, all, or none of the common side effects that have been associated with Rilutek, including:

- Diarrhea
- Dizziness
- Fatigue or drowsiness
- Lightheadedness
- Loss of appetite
- Stomach pain
- Vomiting

- Nausea

Side effects generally go away as your body gets used to the medication. However, if your side effects remain or become worse, consult your doctor to determine if you should continue using the Rilutek. Remember, you should never stop taking your Rilutek or change the dosage without first consulting with your doctor.

Rilutek can also have serious side effects, which are typically rare but of which you should be aware. Serious side effects include:

- Chills
- Cough
- Fever
- A sore throat that does not go away
- A darkening of your urine
- Severe abdominal or stomach pain

If you experience any of those side effects, immediately contact your doctor. Again, severe side effects are rare.

General usage

Your doctor, if he prescribes Rilutek, will advise you on how and when to take it. However, individuals typically take one 50 milligram dose of Rilutek every 12 hours. Of course, the dosage and how often you take the medication will depend on various factors, including your weight.

It is recommended that you take Rilutek either two hours after you have eaten or an hour before you will eat. You should take Rilutek on an empty stomach, unless otherwise instructed by your doctor. Be sure to always follow your doctor's instructions for taking Rilutek; do not intentionally skip doses or change your doses without first consulting your doctor.

Rilutek does not need to be refrigerated but should be kept in a dark area at room temperature.

Estimated cost

Rilutek can be extremely expensive if you do not have health insurance, running around $1,200 a month. However, if you have health insurance or any type of medical coverage, you will probably pay significantly less. Co-pays may range anywhere from twenty dollars to several hundred dollars a month. Your insurance company will be able to tell you how much you can expect to pay, if you have health insurance. You may also be eligible for Medicare, which may cover the Rilutek.

b. Nuedexta

One of the common symptoms of ALS as the disease progresses is a sudden and involuntary emotional outburst. You may, for example, suddenly start crying or laughing uncontrollably. Unfortunately, you have no control over these involuntary outbursts. You may be feeling perfectly content when you start crying. This involuntary outburst, which is common with those who have ALS and MS, is a neurological condition called Involuntary Emotional Expression Disorder (IEED) or Pseudobulbar Affect (PBA).

Doctors will often prescribe the drug Nuedexta to help curb the involuntary expression of emotion. In fact, Nuedexta is used only to treat IEED and is not an anti-depressant. It is also touted as the first medication to treat IEED that has been approved by the Food and Drug Administration.

Side effects

As with any medication, you may experience certain side effects with Nuedexta. However, your doctor will best be able to determine if the benefits will outweigh the potential side effects before prescribing Nuedexta to treat your IEED. Common side effects with Nuedexta include:

- Abnormal liver tests
- Cough
- Diarrhea
- Dizziness
- Flu-like symptoms
- Gas
- General weakness
- Swelling of the ankles or the feet
- Urinary tract infection
- Vomiting

The makers of the drug report that less than 13 percent of patients have experienced side effects when taking Nuedexta. If you experience side effects that persist, contact your doctor. If you have additional side effects not listed, immediately call your doctor.

In rare cases, Nuedexta may cause an abnormal heart rhythm or changes in the rhythm of the heart. If you experience discomfort with your heart or feel an abnormal rhythm in your heart, contact your doctor immediately.

General usage

Your doctor will provide you instructions on how to take the Nuedexta. However, patients, in general, can only take two Nuedexta in a 24 hour period, taking one at 12 hours and another exactly 12 hours later. If you miss a dose, do not take a double dose. Your doctor may prescribe a smaller dose to start, to allow your body to get used to the medication, and to lessen the chances of side effects, before slowly building up to the full daily dose.

You can take Nuedexta with or without food, but it is recommended that you take each dose with a full, eight ounce glass of water and refrain from lying down for at least 10 minutes after taking the medication. Always follow your doctor's instructions for taking the medicine and never make changes, such as suddenly stopping the Nuedexta.

c. Antidepressants

Many people with ALS understandably suffer from anxiety and depression at some point or another during their illness. But, depression and anxiety also affect loved ones, making it important that everyone understands the signs of depression and to know that there is help.

Depression and anxiety can be effectively treated with anti-depressants and/or by talking with a psychologist, as we will discuss in the next chapter, who can help you and your loved ones learn new coping skills.

The good news is depression is not typically severe and does not occur in every one that suffers from ALS, according to the Massachusetts General Hospital, and those who do suffer from depression or anxiety tend to do so shortly after they have been diagnosed rather than later as the disease progresses.

Signs of Depression and Anxiety

Are you or a loved one suffering from depression or anxiety? You may have clinical depression if you have any of the following symptoms and those symptoms have lasted for 14 days or more:

- You have difficulty concentrating.
- You feel hopeless, guilty, or helpless.
- You do not enjoy eating anymore or you just do not have an appetite.
- You have a hard time falling asleep if you wake up in the night.

- You have suicidal thoughts.
- You begin to isolate yourself from your loved ones, preferring to be alone.
- You do not experience pleasure like you used to.
- You are tired even after you have had a good night's sleep of 12 hours.
- Your personality begins to change.

If you have been experiencing any of those symptoms, which persist for two weeks or more, contact your doctor, who may recommend an anti-depressant, a psychologist, or a combination of treatment to help you get back to your normal self.

Anti-depressants for ALS

If your doctor diagnoses you with clinical depression, he is likely to prescribe an anti-depressant to help control your symptoms so you can get back to your normal self. Anti-depressants prescribed to ALS patients are usually done so based on family history with anti-depressants. If a family member has been prescribed an anti-depressant and it worked well for them, the doctor may recommend trying the same medication. In short, there is no specific anti-depressant that doctors prescribe for ALS patients suffering from depression or anxiety.

If you are prescribed an anti-depressant, keep the following in mind:

- You may have to try several different medications to find the one that works for you. Just because one anti-depressant does not work does not mean you stop trying. Your doctor will help you find an anti-depressant that helps manage your symptoms.

- Always take your medication exactly as prescribed by your doctor. As anti-depressants often result in side effects, such as fatigue, your doctor may start you on a lower dose to allow your body to get used to the medicine before gradually working your way up to the full dose.

- Never just stop taking your medication. If you do not feel the anti-depressant is working or the side effects are too much to handle, contact your doctor immediately. Patients must stop taking the anti-depressants slowly. Just as you built up your dosage when you started taking the medication, you will gradually decrease the dosage before you stop taking it altogether. Your doctor will give you exact instructions, which you should follow precisely.

- How quickly your body responds to the anti-depressant really depends. You may begin noticing changes after a few weeks, but it may take a few months for you to start feeling the full affect of the medication.

Most ALS patients taking anti-depressants, according to Massachusetts General Hospital, remain on the medication for approximately six months.

Chapter Six: Treatment: Therapy

If you have been diagnosed with ALS, you are not alone. In addition to a support system of family and friends, you are also likely to work with numerous professionals to help combat the affects of ALS, to help you learn to cope with the changes your body will go through as the disease progresses, to assist you in creating a dietary strategy, and to help you deal with the emotional aspects of ALS.

Among the professionals you may work with now that you have officially been diagnosed with ALS, include:

- A dietitian. As ALS progresses, the muscles in the throat and in the mouth become progressively weaker, making eating difficult and choking and coughing more of a problem. Choking could result in food or liquid going into the lungs, which often leads to respiratory problems, such as pneumonia. A dietitian will make sure you are eating an adequate, nutritious diet with foods that will be less likely to cause choking or coughing.

- An occupational therapist. Now that you have been diagnosed with ALS, you are going to have to make

    changes in your life and in your home to make it easier for you to get around. For example, hand rails in the bath will allow you to safely get in and out of the tub or the shower while you are still able to do so. Ramps in your home will make walking now, and using a wheelchair later on down the road, much easier. An occupational therapist will assess your physical ability and provide you with resources and suggestions for assistive devices, in order to make daily functions easier.

- A physical therapist. Physical therapy, particularly stretching and exercise, is especially important to lessen cramping that is common with ALS and in helping you maintain as much flexibility as possible. The physical therapist, according to the ALS Association of Michigan, will help you maintain your mobility while avoiding fatigue for as long as you are physically able to do so. As the ALS progresses, your physical therapist may also recommended devices, such as a cane, to make walking and moving easier.

- A psychologist. A diagnosis of ALS is extremely difficult and can be an emotional roller coaster for both the person who has been diagnosed and for his or her family and friends. A psychologist can help you and your loved ones deal with your diagnosis and provide you with coping skills and techniques to help you better deal with your emotions. A psychologist will also help you if you develop depression.

- A respiratory therapist. Many people with ALS suffer from respiratory problems, which get worse as the disease progresses. A respiratory therapist can recommend a breathing mask or a ventilator, when necessary, and can offer suggestions on how to conserve energy.

- A speech pathologist. One of the early signs of ALS is slurred speech or a difficulty in projecting one's voice. A speech pathologist will work with you on both your speech and your swallowing issues, offering recommendations for speech generating devices, for how to communicate non-verbally, and for how to deal with difficulty swallowing.

Now that you have an idea of the help various professionals can provide, let's take a look at the different forms of therapy available and how you may benefit from each.

a. Occupational Therapy

Upon your ALS diagnosis, your doctor is likely to recommend that you see an occupational therapist who will help you learn how to live with Lou Gehrig's Disease by adapting your lifestyle, your car, and your home to make every day activities easier, especially as the disease progresses. Occupational therapists will:

- Assess how well your arms function.

- Walk through your home, offering specific recommendations – such as chair lifts for the stairs, ramps, and rails in the bathroom – to make your home more accessible and easier for you to maneuver around.

- Provide you with ideas on how to conserve your energy and make everyday tasks easier.

- Determine when you will need to begin using an assistive device for walking, such as a walker, and decide what type of wheelchair you will need before you actually need to use it. The occupational therapist will also teach you how to use a walker or a wheelchair so that you can safely move around.

- Train your caregiver(s) on how to care for you. For example, the occupational therapist will show your caregiver how to move you from your wheelchair, when applicable, into your bed or onto the couch in a way that you do not become injured.

In Chapter Eight, we will discuss in-depth the many assistive living devices your occupational therapist may recommend to help you maintain your independence and your mobility.

Learn how to use a wheelchair

At some point, you will need to use a wheelchair to be able to move around. An occupational therapist will help you plan for using a wheelchair now. A customized wheelchair is just that: It is customized to your body and to your needs. As a result, you cannot just order a wheelchair and expect it to be ready tomorrow or even next week.

Your occupational therapist will discuss using a wheelchair with you before you ever need it. You can then order it and it will be ready when you are ready to start using it.

Once you have your wheelchair, your occupational therapist will teach you how to use it.

b. Physical Therapy

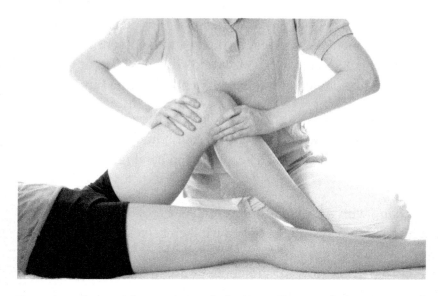

Exercise plays an important role in every human being's mental and physical wellbeing. It is perhaps even more important if you have ALS. In addition to keeping your spirits up, exercise will help you maintain a sense of independence. Most experts recommend ALS patients exercise for as long as they are physically able.

Your doctor may recommend you make an appointment with a physical therapist soon after your diagnosis to begin treatment. Your physical therapist will assess your level of flexibility and range of motion and, based on those results, will recommend gentle exercises and stretching techniques. The physical therapist will teach you the exercises and will provide you with printouts showing you exactly what to do when she is not there.

A physical therapist may also recommend, depending on your mobility, water exercises and biking.

In addition, a physical therapist can recommend, when it is necessary, using a cane, ankle braces, or a walker. Caregivers also receive assistance from physical therapists. If you are a caregiver, the physical therapist will teach you how to help your loved one with stretching and other exercises and will show you how to move your loved one without inadvertently injuring him or her.

Some physical therapists also provide home assessments, much like occupational therapists, visiting your home and assessing ways to make mobility, such as ramps and hand rails, easier and safer.

Exercising with ALS is far different than exercising before your diagnosis. Many healthy people push themselves to their physical limits when they exercise. You, however, have to be careful with exercising. When you are stretching or doing exercises your physical therapist recommended, keep the following in mind:

- Do not push yourself to the point of extreme fatigue. Even if you are having a really good day and feel like you can take on the world, you are likely to feel the effects of pushing yourself too hard later in the day or the next day.

- Not sure if you are pushing yourself too hard? Are you tired and sore from your workout the next day? If you are tired and sore the next day, you are working too hard. Pull back a little bit.

- Plan your exercise around your daily activities. You are going to tire much more quickly now that you have ALS, so it is important to make sure you have adequate time to rest between your daily activities and exercise.

c. Benefits of Exercise

Not everyone enjoys exercising, but it should become a new habit in your life as long as you are able to exercise. You will find that there are numerous benefits to exercising, such as:

- Exercise often helps lessen incidents of muscle spasms. Muscle spasms are a common symptom of ALS and can be very painful.

- Those with ALS experience a permanent tightening of their muscles and exercise may help slow the progression of that permanent tightening.

- Exercise has proven to help relieve the symptoms of depression and is recommended to help maintain good physical and mental wellbeing.

d. Finding a Qualified Physical Therapist

You must find a physical therapist who has experience working with ALS patients. An experienced physical therapist will know how the disease progresses and will know which exercises work best for each stage of ALS.

To find a qualified physical therapist:

1. Ask your neurologist or doctor if he can recommend a physical therapist.

2. Contact your local branch of the ALS Association.

3. Consult the American Physical Therapy Association. You can plug in your city and zip code, the specialty for which you are looking (neurology), and you will be given a page of results.

e. Conserving Energy

Regardless of where you are with ALS, you will need to conserve your energy. Fatigue is a common part of life with ALS and it can sometimes be overwhelming. As you learn to live with ALS, you will also find ways to conserve energy and to make things easier on you. Here are several simple ideas that will help you from becoming overexerted and will help you save energy:

- Use warm water when taking a bath or a shower. Water that is too hot or too cold could make you very tired.

- If you prefer showers to baths, purchase a shower stool so you can sit while you shower.

- Apply for a handicap permit. Even if you are no longer able to drive, your caregiver can apply for a handicap permit to make it easier for you when you go out in public. The further you have to walk, the more tired you will become, and you do not want to wear yourself out before you even get out of the parking lot. To apply for a handicap sticker, you will generally have to fill out a form from the Department of Motor Vehicles in your state and have your doctor verify your need for it.

- Steer clear of stress. Everyone has stress in their lives, but do your best to avoid situations that will cause you stress.

Stress can lead to fatigue.

- Be aware of how your body reacts to extreme heat or cold. Some people with ALS become fatigued after spending time or exerting themselves while in the heat or the cold. Do not push yourself in extreme temperatures.

- Use assistive devices that will make your life easier.

- Pace yourself. If you become tired walking from the living room to the kitchen, walk a few steps then take a break to catch your breath to prevent overexerting yourself.

- Make your environment more convenient for you. Your bedroom may not have a bathroom, so you have to get up and walk to go to the bathroom. Your child's bedroom may be right next door to the bathroom. Instead of tiring yourself out, consider having someone rearrange the bedrooms for you. If you are sitting in your favorite chair in the living room and normally have to get up to answer the phone, bring the phone closer to you. Arrange your living space so it is more convenient for you.

- Consume enough calories daily. Researchers have found that those who were overweight or at their normal weight at the time of diagnosis fared better against the disease than those who were underweight at the time of diagnosis or who rapidly lost weight upon being told they had ALS. Do your best to avoid losing weight and to get the nutrition you need each day.

- Go to bed at the same time each night and get up around the same time each day. Establishing a routine can help ensure you get the rest you need each day.

As you move forward, you will find other ways to make your life easier so you can conserve energy. Do whatever is necessary to ensure that you do not overexert yourself.

f. Speech Therapy

One of the early signs of Lou Gehrig's Disease is slurred speech. As the ALS progresses, the muscles in the mouth and in the throat begin to weaken, which leads to difficulty or an inability to speak or to swallow without assistance. Speech therapists or speech pathologists provide individuals with ALS with assistance with both speaking and with swallowing issues, which we will discuss in the next section.

Speaking

A speech therapist can help you learn how to communicate both verbally and non-verbally, the latter of which can help you to preserve precious energy. Experts recommend several techniques to allow you to effectively communicate without causing too much stress on your muscles. It is important to remember that when you are tired at the end of the day, you will also have more trouble speaking.

To preserve energy and to effectively communicate, you can do the following:

- Face the person with whom you are speaking. Even in the early stages of ALS, you may have difficulty projecting your voice, which could make it hard for others to hear you. Look at the person you are talking to to help make communicating easier.

- Eliminate outside noises, when possible. If you are having difficulty projecting your voice, you are not going to be able to compete with a television or a radio on in the background. Try to hold conversations in a relatively quiet atmosphere.

- Consult your speech therapist before starting any new exercises designed to help your speaking. You may read about exercises you can do to help strengthen your muscles. Those exercises could, however, simply cause you to become more tired, faster and work against your goal of being able to speak better. Discuss viable

  exercise options with your speech pathologist before adding new exercises to your routine.

- Talk slowly, using short phrases. Choose your words carefully, so you do not have to speak as long, thus allowing you to preserve energy.

- Only start speaking when you have the other person's attention. The Les Turner ALS Foundation recommends having a signal to those people with whom you communicate, so they know when you want to say something.

- Take your time when speaking. If you need to pause between phrases or even between words, do so. Rushing through the conversation is likely to tire you out much faster.

- Plan your conversations. While it is not always possible to plan when you are going to speak, sometimes you can. If you know a friend is going to call or you have to call your doctor's office, for example, make sure you rest your voice and conserve your energy before your conversation. As ALS progresses, even speaking can tire you out.

- Write down what you want to say. Before the ALS progresses and you can no longer write without a lot of effort, you may want to carry around a pad and a pen to write down whatever you want to say, if the other person does not understand you. As the ALS progresses, your speech pathologist may recommended using a tool, such as an alphabet board or a speech generating device, that will help you get your message across.

- Use hand gestures and facial gestures for as long as you still can. You may be too tired to talk or to continue a conversation. Sometimes a facial expression or a hand gesture can allow you to effectively get your point across without you having to exert energy by speaking.

If your loved one has ALS, be patient and remember that he will no longer be able to speak as quickly or as loudly as he once could. Even simple conversations may take significantly longer and your loved one may become frustrated. Offer your support and remain patient.

Speech Assistive Devices

Your speech pathologist may recommend speech assistive devices that can help you with communicating. Devices that are available to those with ALS include:

Alphabet Board

An alphabet board is similar to using a pen and paper and is ideal if you cannot write as well as you used to. An alphabet board is a board with all the letters of the alphabet and may also contain certain commonly used words. You simply point to the letters on the board to spell out the message you are trying to communicate.

Some individuals with ALS become creative and, in addition to using an alphabet or a letter board, have created their own picture boards. For example, if you want to use the bathroom but are too fatigued to speak, you simply need to point to the picture of the toilet. If you are thirsty, you might point to a picture of a filled glass.

You can find various types of communicative boards through Low Tech Solutions.

Palatal Lift

A palatal lift is comparable to a retainer and is generally recommended for those with ALS who have nasal issues when speaking. The palatal lift, which lifts your soft palate, is designed to prevent air from going out of the nose while you are wearing it. ALS patients are fitted for a palatal lift by going to a prosthodontist. Over the course of several visits, the prosthodontist will measure and fit the palatal lift. Palatal lifts are generally not recommended for ALS patients whose speech muscles, including the tongue, are rapidly becoming weaker.

Record Your Voice: "Voice Banking"

If you still have a strong voice, you may want to record your voice so you can use it later. Voice banking, according to Massachusetts General Hospital, requires that you read specific words and phrases into an audio system, usually on a computer. Your words are then created into a computerized communication device. When you have lost the ability to communicate verbally, you will enter words or specific phrases into the computer, which will then be read back in your voice. Model Talker is one company that offers a voice banking system, which will allow you to record your voice now so you can use it again in the future.

TTY Telephone Device

A TTY telephone device may not be necessary if you have a voice amplifier or a speaking device that allows you to speak loud and clear. However, a TTY telephone device is helpful for those with ALS or with other speech problems who need to use the telephone. Instead of talking into the phone, you will have a keyboard in which you can text the message you want to convey. The catch with the TTY is you either have to speak to someone else who has the device, so he or she can read what you have written. Or, you can contact the operator who will relay the message for you.

If you use the phone a lot but have a lot of difficulty speaking, ask your speech pathologist if a TTY might be an ideal solution.

Voice Amplifier

Some people with ALS have difficulty projecting their voices, making it hard for others to hear them when they speak. If you speak softly or have trouble projecting your voice, your speech therapist may recommend a voice amplifier. A voice amplifier will do what you cannot: Make your voice louder so others can hear you when you speak.

The voice amplifier is a small speaker with a wire attached to it. The speaker portion of the voice amplifier can be held on your lap or attached to your waist with a band. The second part of the voice amplifier is the microphone, which you can attach to your shirt. The microphone can also be attached to a headset to make it easier to use.

A voice amplifier only makes your voice louder. As a result, if your speech is not clear, the device is not going to be much of a help. Your speech pathologist may recommend a voice amplifier if you become fatigued from trying to speak so others can hear you and if you still maintain clarity of your speech.

Voice amplifiers are an ideal option, especially when you go to noisy places such as a restaurant with customers talking and music playing.

Will Your Insurance Cover An Assistive Device?

A speech pathologist will evaluate you and help determine the best communicative devices for your needs. You must be evaluated by a speech pathologist, which is generally covered under most insurance plans, before you can even think about getting a communication assistive device. Be sure that whatever speech therapist you engage for your evaluation has extensive knowledge of ALS and has worked with ALS patients before. Your speech pathologist must understand how your needs will change as the ALS progresses.

Once the speech pathologist assesses your needs, he or she will recommend an appropriate device or devices. That is when you will have to determine how you will pay for the device: through Medicare or private insurance, and if you do not have private insurance, how you can afford the devices you need to make your life easier.

The ALS Association of Philadelphia asserts that ALS patients with Medicare B generally have the cost of "Speech Generating Devices" or SGDs covered under their Medicare plan. However, to be eligible for Medicare B, you must still live at home or must be currently living in an assisted living facility. Medicare B is not available for those people receiving hospice care, living in a nursing facility, or currently in the hospital.

Generally, Medicare will cover 80 percent of the necessary speech generating devices, which means your health insurance, if you have it, will have to cover the rest. If your insurance does not cover the additional 20 percent, you may have to pay out of pocket or you can contact your local ALS Association or your doctor to determine if there are funding assistance programs available to you.

Health Insurance

Whether your health insurance, if you have it, will cover the cost of a speech generating device really depends upon your individual plan.

The ALS Association of Philadelphia recommends that ALS patients contact their health insurance providers and request that they be assigned a case manager. A case manager will get to know your case and will be able to help you navigate through the red tape that is often required to get approval for an assistive device. A case manager will also help you file claims, answer any questions you may have, and advocate on your behalf.

Contact your health insurance company to determine the process for obtaining a case manager. You may simply only have to request one, or your doctor may have to call on your behalf and request a case manager be assigned to your case.

No Insurance

Unfortunately, not everyone in the United States has health insurance. And, in some cases, even if they do have health insurance, that insurance does not cover speech generating devices. If you do not have health insurance or your health insurance does not cover the speech generating device, you have several options for getting the equipment you need.

- The ALS Association has branches throughout the United States, and you may be able to borrow a speech generating device from your local branch of the ALS Association.

- Contact the manufacturer of the speech generating device to determine if you can rent a device.

- You can generally purchase the speech generating device directly from the manufacturer. Purchasing the device yourself, especially if you are going to be using it quite frequently, can be beneficial in that it is yours to keep.

You do not have to return it and no one else but you will use it.

Do not be discouraged if your health insurance does not cover a speech generating device. Remember, you still have options for getting the equipment you need. Your speech pathologist may also be able to recommend resources that offer financial assistance.

Swallowing

As ALS progresses and the muscles in the mouth, the tongue, and the throat begin to significantly weaken, people have difficulty chewing and swallowing food. Choking and coughing can result in severe problems, especially as the ALS progresses. If you aspirate food into your lungs, you may develop pneumonia or other respiratory illnesses.

A speech pathologist will help you through every stage of the ALS, starting with an evaluation process to determine how well you are currently swallowing. The evaluation is nothing to worry about and generally consists of the speech pathologist watching as you drink a glass of water or eat a small piece of food, such as a cookie or a cracker.

The speech pathologist will watch to see if you experience coughing or choking, if food or water dribbles out of the sides of your mouth, and whether or not you have difficulty swallowing. If the speech pathologist is concerned about your swallowing, she may request that you complete a Modified Barium Swallow or MBS.

The MBS is performed by both your speech pathologist and a radiologist, who performs X-rays. The test is simple and painless. You will be given small amount of liquid and food, each with a different consistency, and asked to swallow each. Tiny traces of barium are contained in everything you digest. The X-ray machine then shows what happens when you eat and drink different foods and liquids.

An MBS allows a speech pathologist to better assess what is going on and can offer suggestions to make swallowing easier for you. Your diet will play a key role throughout the rest of your life. Even in the beginning, when you may not be experiencing any problems with swallowing, your speech pathologist will emphasize the importance of eating a balanced, healthy diet. As the ALS progresses, your speech pathologist will offer assistance on the types of food you should eat and their consistency to ensure you are getting the proper nutrients with minimal chances of choking or coughing.

g. Respiratory Therapy

Many people with ALS deal with breathing problems, as a result of weakening muscles in the respiratory system, which requires some form of intervention. However, you may not even realize you are starting to have problems with your breathing at first. The ALS Association of Michigan cites several common symptoms that may signal you are having trouble breathing, including:

- You begin having trouble sleeping but cannot pinpoint a reason for your inability to sleep.

- You wake up with a headache in the morning.

- You do not sleep as well lying down in bed as you do sitting up in a chair or in a recliner.

- You need more than one or two pillows to comfortably sleep.

- You begin coughing more.

- You just feel more tired than usual.

If you start experiencing any of those symptoms, the ALS Association of Michigan recommends calling your doctor to make an appointment for a respiratory evaluation, which will tell you if an assistive breathing device is necessary.

Respiratory Breathing Device

You generally have two options when it comes to using a respiratory assistive device: Non-invasive, such as a breathing mask, and invasive, which requires doctors to insert a hole in your trachea.

A Bi-Level Positive Air Pressure, or BIPAP, provides non-invasive breathing assistance for those with ALS. Essentially, the BIPAP does the breathing for you.

Most ALS patients begin using a BIPAP at night when they sleep and, as their muscles become progressively weaker, start using it all of the time. You generally have three options with the BIPAP: a mask that covers your nose, a face mask that covers your entire face, or a nasal pillow, which are essentially little cushions you put in your nose.

Your doctor is more likely to recommend a BIPAP once you have a breathing capacity of less than 50 percent.

Some people with ALS use a ventilator, which is an invasive approach. A ventilator is a machine that does all of your breathing for you, and you will generally have to be hooked up to it all of the time. With a ventilator, you will have a tracheostomy, which means the doctors will create a hole in your trachea and a tube will be inserted through the hole. The tube may be metal or plastic.

A ventilator will change your life drastically in that you will no longer be able to be left alone and will need around the clock care from a nurse or another medical professional. Your caregiver may also be trained in how to care for you and to ensure the ventilator is always working properly.

The good news with a ventilator is that you can remain at home, although some people with ALS opt to go into a nursing home for the required care associated with the ventilator and the progression of the ALS. It is important to note that the ventilator is only designed to assist you in breathing better. It cannot stop the progression of the ALS or reverse it in any way.

Deciding whether or not to use a ventilator is a very personal decision. You may decide that a ventilator will help extend your life, especially if you are coping well with your ALS. If your ALS has progressed to the point where you are severely disabled or you have extreme difficulty communicating, you may not want to use a ventilator.

If you choose to use a ventilator, you should be aware that your ability to speak may be affected. Talk with your respiratory therapist about the benefits and the downsides of using a ventilator. If you are living at home, you will also have to consider who is going to provide care for you. Will your insurance cover a nurse or another medical professional? Will your caregiver take on some of the responsibility for learning how to care for you with a ventilator? If so, who will care for you while she is on a break? Is she willing to sacrifice much of her own life to care for your needs?

Again, consult with your doctor and make the decision with your caregiver. Some people with ALS, who have opted to use a ventilator, have gone on to live for many years.

Respiratory Care Tips

Respiratory problems are a very real problem for those with ALS, requiring some patients to use masks to assist with breathing while others may need to have a hole inserted into the trachea for a ventilator to allow for easier breathing. In addition to therapy, you can take some steps to help avoid respiratory problems, including:

- Do your best to avoid family and friends with a cold or the flu, so you do not, too, become sick and risk further complications, such as pneumonia.

- Take preventative measures to avoid getting sick, such as getting an annual flu shot and any other vaccinations your doctor recommends.

- Rather than eating three large meals a day, eat smaller meals more frequently each day.

- Avoid lying down immediately after you eat. The ALS Association recommends that you remain in an upright position for a minimum of an hour following meals.

h. Alternative Treatments

Some people with ALS, in addition to traditional medication and treatments, seek alternative options for relieving their symptoms of ALS and in an attempt to slow the progression of the disease. Alternative therapies are classified as such because there is no evidence that the treatment works and most doctors recommend a traditional course of treatment and therapy.

The ALS Research Group defines alternative therapy as "Treatments for which there is no good evidence that patients with ALS use instead of or in addition to treatments that are proven and recommended by ALS experts."

Essentially, doctors and other medical professionals do not recommend alternative therapy although two in particular, acupuncture and Chelation, seem to be popular among some people with ALS.

Red Flags with Potential Alternative Treatments for ALS

Before you decide to try an alternative treatment, be sure that you do your proper research first about the company offering the treatment and be aware of the red flags that more often than not signify you are dealing with a scam. Common red flags include:

- You are promised a cure. Researchers have spent decades working to find the cause of and a cure for Lou Gehrig's Disease. To date, there is no cure. Any alternative treatment or medication that promises to cure ALS is untrue. If such a miracle treatment existed, it would be all over the news.

- The company or individual offering the treatment insists that proof that it works exists and offers client testimonials as proof. Again, if a treatment worked it would be widely discussed in the media and your doctor would recommend you try it.

- Your insurance will not pay for the treatment. While insurance not paying for the treatment is not a sure sign of a scam, it should send up red flags. Consult with your doctor.

- You must pay for the treatment by sending a large sum of money overseas.

Acupuncture

Many people claim that acupuncture is a great form of therapy for many illnesses and diseases, including ALS. While acupuncture does not reverse the affects of ALS nor does it slow the progression of the disease, some people with ALS have found that it can alleviate some of their symptoms for the short-term.

Before trying acupuncture or any form of treatment, be sure to consult with your doctor. You may also want to discuss the effects – both good and bad – that those with ALS have experienced when trying acupuncture. An online discussion board or a forum is the ideal place to find those who have tried acupuncture and, if you are a member of a support group that meets in person, talk with others to determine if they have tried acupuncture.

Chelation

Chelation works on the premise that ALS is caused by heavy metals, including lead. EDTA Chelation therapy is generally used to combat the effects of heavy metal poisoning. A substance called EDTA removes the heavy metals from the body during therapy. Because some people believe that ALS may be caused by heavy metals, they opt for the Chelation therapy. Chelation therapy may be given orally or intravenously.

Those who receive Chelation therapy intravenously have to go to the doctor's office or medical facility several times a week to receive the therapy, which is typically ongoing, and generally costs several hundreds of dollars per session. Contact your insurance company to determine if the treatment will be covered.

The potential side effects of Chelation therapy, according to the ALS Research Group, include:

- Kidney failure
- An allergic reaction
- Respiratory problems and failure
- Abnormal heart beat

If you are interested in Chelation therapy or any alternative therapies, discuss them with your doctor first, so you have a full understanding of the potential risks and benefits.

Chapter Seven: Making Every Day Life Easier

Individuals with ALS must adapt their everyday living to cope with the progression of the disease. Everyday tasks – such as eating and dressing oneself – become increasingly harder as the body's muscles begin to weaken. As the disease progresses, most people will ALS must learn how to communicate without the use of their voice, must learn how to move around after losing their ability to walk, and must learn how to eat a proper diet that is easy to swallow.

Fortunately, there are many assistive devices that may help you during each stage of the disease. Even better, many insurance companies and Medicare often cover, at least in part, such expensive assistive devices as speech generating devices and eye gazing technology.

Invest some time, if you have it, to find out what other people are saying about the devices you are considering purchasing. Go on support and other ALS forums and request feedback. You will also discover many other ideas that those with ALS and their loved ones have used that can also help you and your loved ones adapt to life with ALS.

a. Speech Generating Devices

As ALS begins to progress, you may no longer be able to use your hands and may no longer be able to speak. Eye gazing technology allows those with ALS to control the computer screen on a speech generating device using only their eye movements, which are tracked by a camera. Most eye gazing technology allows individuals with ALS to use the computer as normal, including going online and checking emails.

Be sure to purchase the eye gazing technology while you or your loved one is still doing relatively well, as many who have used the eye gaze say it takes time and practice to get used to using. It is generally for those who have little to no use of their hands and may be covered by private insurance and/or Medicare.

You can find speech generating devices using eye gazing technology through numerous companies, including:

- LC Technologies: http://eyegaze.com/eyegaze-assistive-technology-products/

- DynaVox: http://www.dynavoxtech.com/products/eyemax/

- Tobii: http://www.tobii.com/en/assistive-technology/global/

- Boundless Assistive Technology: http://www.boundlessat.com/Communication/Speech-Generating-Devices

Your doctor, speech pathologist, or occupational therapist may be able to offer additional recommendations of companies that sell speech generating devices using eye gazing technology.

b. Food Thickener

Your dietitian or speech pathologist may recommend that you eat foods with a certain consistency to make swallowing easier and to prevent coughing or choking. You may be able to puree food, or you can also try one of the food thickeners on the market, such as Thick-it.

Thick-it sells pureed food, food thickeners, and beverages specifically for people who have swallowing problems. The company's products are sold online and in such stores as Walgreen's, Rite Aid, CVS, and Walmart. To learn more about Thick-it products and how to order, visit their website at http://www.thickitretail.com/.

Your speech pathologist or dietitian may also be able to recommend specific products to use or ways to make your food easier to swallow.

c. Walkers/Wheelchairs

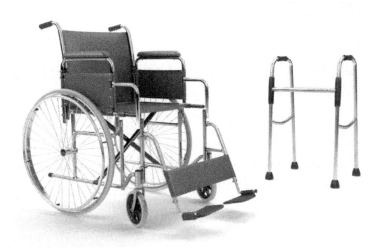

As you begin to have difficulty walking, your occupational therapist will probably recommend that you start to use a walker. (Canes are generally not safe for those with ALS, making the individual prone to falling). A walker will allow you to maintain your mobility and keep your muscles active. As pushing the walker becomes more difficult, you can put wheels on your walker or purchase a walker with wheels.

Your occupational therapist, as we discussed earlier, will talk with you about using a wheelchair long before you ever need one. A customized wheelchair takes time to build and you will not have to wait for your wheelchair when you need it if you order it early.

d. Chair Lifts/Other Lifts

Chair lifts allow for going up and down the stairs without having to walk. You sit down on a chair, push a button on a remote control, and the chair lift slowly takes you up or down the stairs. Lifts are also available to lift a wheelchair into a van or a truck. Among the companies that sell chair lifts include:

- All Chair Lifts: http://www.chairliftmusic.com/

- AmeriGlide: http://www.ameriglide.com/wheelchair

- Bruno Independent Living Aids: http://www.bruno.com/bruno-all-products.html

- Silver Cross (Recycled & New Healthcare Equipment; does not sell chair lifts but provides information on chair lifts, including how to choose the best chair lift):

http://www.silvercross.com/stairlifts.html

- ThyssenKrupp Access Solutions:
  http://www.tkaccess.com/

Many communities also have medical supply stores that sell living aids, including chair lifts. Check online, your local phone book, or ask your doctor or a member of your medical team if they know of a local company that sells medical supplies and living aids.

e. Ramps

As your ALS progresses, you will begin to lose your ability to walk, eventually requiring a wheelchair. Ramps inside and outside of your home will make getting around possible. Some companies also sell portable wheelchair ramps. You can purchase, or may be able to rent, wheelchair ramps for your home at companies such as:

- American Access, Inc.: http://www.aaramps.com/

- Express Ramps: http://www.portable-wheelchair

- EZ Access: http://ezaccess.com

- Hoveround: http://www.hoveround.com/power-chair-accessories/wheelchair

- Walgreen's (portable wheelchair ramps):
  http://www.walgreens.com/q/portable-wheelchair

f. Wrist/Hand/Leg Brace

As your mobility becomes compromised, your occupational therapist or another member of your medical team may recommend getting a wrist, hand, or leg brace to help support you in moving around. If you are getting a leg brace, for example, you will generally have to be fitted for it and your doctor or medical professional will probably order it for you. Discuss braces with your occupational therapist as you notice your muscles in your wrist, hands, and legs begin to weaken.

g. Making Life Easier

In addition to assistive devices you can use to make life easier, you can also do some simple things to make everyday living more comfortable in all stages of ALS, including:

- Replace the buttons and zippers on clothes with Velcro to make getting dressed and undressed easier for both the person with ALS and the caregiver.

- Wear shirts you just have to pull over your head and pants or shorts you just have to pull up (and do not have buttons or zippers), especially in the early part of the disease when you still have some normal use of your fingers and your hands.

- Use a shoe horn with a long handle to make it easier to put shoes on.

- Wear slip-on shoes instead of shoes with ties.

- Purchase a shower chair that you can slide across to get in and out of the shower.

- Install a handheld shower head to allow you to effectively and easily bathe your loved one.

- A raised toilet seat can help with getting on and off of the toilet in the early stages of the disease.

- Replace your light switches. If you have the traditional switches that require you to push up or down to turn the light on or off, change them for switches that simply require you to gently touch them to turn the light on or off.

- To avoid getting your loved one's clothes soaked when you wash his hair, drape a lightweight poncho over him.

- Install a walk-in shower in your bathroom to make it easier, especially as the ALS progresses.

- Move the bars in your closets lower, making it easier to remove clothes and other items, especially when you still have mobility.

- Recliners are available that allow you to push a button on a remote, which will elevate you into the standing position and vice-versa.

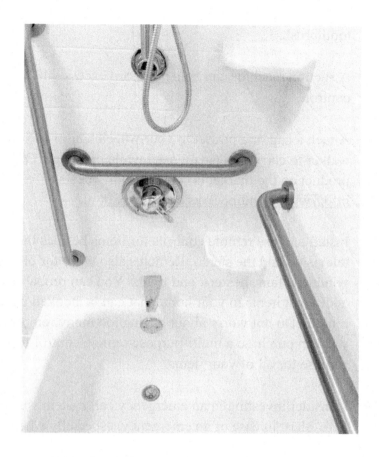

- Install hand rails in your bathroom's tub or shower. Rails are also available for toilets, which allow you to hold on as you stand up and sit down.

- Use dry shampoo to wash your loved one's hair.

- Purchase a portable urinal, which you may have to help your loved one use.

- Opt for an electric toothbrush instead of a manual toothbrush.

- A suction machine can help you keep excess saliva under control.

- Attach a bag or a pocket to your wheelchair or to your walker to carry things you need while on the go. One product on the market is called HandiPockets: http://www.handipockets.com/index.html.

- Install and use remote controls for items besides the television and the stereo. Remotes also work for blinds on windows, fans, heaters, and lights. You can probably find additional items in your home that can be hooked up to a remote. Do not worry about having too many remotes as you can purchase a multi-purpose remote control that you can use for all of your items.

- Consider investing in an emergency call system, such as Life Alert, in case of an emergency, especially when

  you are alone in the early stages of ALS. You generally wear such a product around your neck or on your wrist.

- Listen to audio books on your MP3 player or your iPod when you can no longer hold or turn the pages of a book.

- Use voice recognition software to assist you in using your computer while your voice is still clear. If your word processing package does not come with voice recognition software, you can purchase software like Dragon Speech Recognition Software. The software does all of the work for you – typing, checking your email, and going online – all by the sound of your voice.

h. Other Resources

Many companies offer assistive devices and aids. Following are several resources that may help as you look for ways to adapt your life and your home to ALS:

- Seating Solutions, Inc. offers a full list of different companies that sell products for those with ALS. You

  can check out their products and resources page at: http://www.seatingsolutionsinc.com/index.php/products-organizations/.

- The ALS Association also offers an extensive list of products available to help those with ALS at: http://www.alsa.org/als-care/resources/products/.

- Ablenet.com sells assistive devices for those with ALS: http://www.ablenetinc.com/Assistive-Technology/Applications-of-AT/ALS-Lou-Gehrigs-Disease

- Permobil allows visitors to view a video created by the ALS Association and lists an extensive list of products available for those with ALS: http://countries.permobil.com/USA/Products/Support/ALS-Support-Video/

Chapter Eight: Financial Considerations

In addition to the emotional and physical aspects of a diagnosis of Lou Gehrig's Disease, most people also have to deal with the financial considerations of dealing with all that is required to care for a loved one with ALS, especially as the disease progresses and more care and equipment will be needed to maintain comfort and everyday living. Your loved one will have no choice but to stop working, either now or eventually, which could put an additional burden on your finances.

The overwhelming costs of caring for someone with ALS can be quite stressful, especially if you are like many people and do not have health insurance coverage. The good news is you are not alone and there are many options for caring for your loved one. Following are some options you may be able to use to help pay for the costs of Lou Gehrig's Disease.

a. Ask for a Case Manager

As we already discussed in Chapter Seven, contact your health insurance company – or have your doctor do so on your behalf, if necessary – and ask that your loved one's health insurance policy be assigned a case manager. A case manager will become familiar with your case, will be able to answer any questions you may have about coverage, and will become your loved one's advocate.

b. Apply for Medicaid

Americans in the low income bracket are generally eligible for Medicaid coverage. Medicaid provides medical coverage to those individuals who cannot otherwise afford it, provided they meet such eligibility requirements as income that falls below the poverty line. Individuals applying for Medicaid will also have to provide a list of their assets in addition to their monthly income to determine eligibility.

Medicaid also offers a retroactive period. If you did not apply for Medicaid but were eligible for it at least three months prior to your application, you can receive coverage for those three months once your coverage begins. If you are no longer eligible to receive Medicaid, your medical coverage will cease that same month.

c. Apply for Medicare

Medicare is immediately available for those with ALS, according to the Center for Medical Advocacy, Inc., as soon as the individual begins receiving social security disability payments. Medicare generally provides partial or full coverage for hospital stays, doctor's visits, necessary equipment, and home health care.

You can call 1-800-MEDICARE for more information and to apply.

d. Apply for Social Security Disability

For every paycheck you have earned in your life in the United States, you have had a percentage withdrawn for social security. Generally, you will begin accessing those funds when you retire at the age of 65. A diagnosis of ALS will allow you to immediately begin receiving social security disability payments, provided you have met the work guidelines, according to the ALS Association of St. Louis.

SSI benefits are also available for those who have been diagnosed with ALS and who are qualified as lower income. If you are qualified for Medicaid, you are generally also eligible for SSI benefits.

To determine if you are eligible for social security disability or to apply for social security, go to http://www.ssa.gov/. You can apply online or by calling 1-800-772-1213.

e. Consult a Tax Professional

A good tax professional can provide you with invaluable advice on what medical and other expenses you can claim as deductions on your taxes. Be sure to keep all of your receipts for medical expenses and other expenses related to the ALS.

f. Fundraising

Fundraising is a popular and an effective way of raising money for the specific needs of your loved one with ALS. For example, perhaps you do not have the necessary funds to purchase a customized wheelchair or to have your home modified to make it easier for your loved one to get around. Family and friends of loved ones with illnesses, such as ALS or cancer, often throw fundraisers to raise money to pay for such needs. Fundraising ideas might include:

- Hosting dinners with all profits going to your loved one.

- Holding mini-marathons or walks with participants raising pledges for every mile they walk.

- Having bake sales or hoagie sales.

- Holding yard sales.

One little girl, who was fighting an aggressive form of brain cancer, made crafts that her family then sold online to help pay for her ongoing care. Her mom also ran a blog and a Facebook page that allowed people, many of whom became emotionally invested and learned much about the illness that later claimed her life, to follow the family's journey. Fundraising ideas are really only limited by your imagination.

g. Downsize

You may be required to downsize your life to save money. Moving into a smaller home might not be an option, especially with all that you now have to deal with, but what about your car? Perhaps you are driving a new car. Selling it and driving an older model could cut down on monthly car payments. Opting for basic cable over expanded cable and purchasing lesser known brands instead of the more popular, expensive brands are all ways to cut costs and save money as you find ways to financially manage your loved one's ALS expenses.

h. Contact the Manufacturer

If your health insurance does not cover equipment or you do not have health insurance, contact the manufacturer of the equipment to determine if you can rent it for as long as necessary. Likewise, if you cannot afford to pay for expensive medications, try contacting the drug's manufacturer to see if they have a financial assistance program or can provide you with the medication at a discounted price.

Chapter Nine: Should You Participate in a Clinical Trial?

a. What is a Clinical Trial?

The National Institutes of Health defines clinical trials, which are integral to finding a cure for Lou Gehrig's Disease, as "one type of clinical research that follows a pre-defined plan or protocol. By taking part in clinical trials, participants can not only play a more active role in their own health care, but they can also access new treatments and help others by contributing to medical research."

Clinical trials, according to the National Institutes of Health, are conducted in three phases:

- Phase one includes a small group of participants who are recruited to test an innovative treatment or drug. Researchers are testing to determine the overall safety of the treatment or the drug, the safest dosage range for medications, and the potential side effects of the treatment.

- Phase two of the clinical trial involves a much larger group of participants, which allows researchers to determine if the drug or the treatment is effective in a larger group of people and to again assess whether the drug or the treatment is safe.

- Phase three allows researchers to evaluate the treatment or medication even further by giving it to numerous large groups of people. In the third phase, researchers will assess the effectiveness of the treatment or the medication and keep track of the side effects the participants experience. Researchers will also compare its effectiveness to other treatments already on the market.

- Phase four occurs once the treatment or medication has been introduced to the public. Researchers initiate studies to determine how the medication or treatment is working among different segments of the population and to assess whether there are any side effects that result when the medication or treatment is used long-term.

Clinical trials evaluate treatments and medications for all illnesses and diseases including ALS, cancer, depression, diabetes, fibromyalgia, and chronic pain. In the third section,

"How to find Clinical Trials," you will find resources for finding an ALS clinical trial for which you may be eligible.

b. ALS-related Clinical trials

Researchers have spent decades trying to pinpoint the exact causes of ALS and how to reverse or to cure the effects of the disease. Clinical trials play an important part in that research.

Participating in a clinical trial will allow you to contribute to the research that could lead to answers as to how to better treat ALS. However, you really have to consider whether you want to participate in a clinical trial and how it will impact your own life. To assess whether participating in a clinical trial is right for you, talk with the trial's coordinator and ask plenty of questions, such as:

- Do I fit the eligibility requirements for the clinical trial(s) in which I am interested?

- What are the potential risks of the treatment or the medication being studied?

- What are the potential benefits of the treatment or the medication?

- Will I still be able to take my medications and continue the course of treatment I am on?

- How much time will be required of me?

- Will I still be able to participate in my normal activities while I am a participant in the trial?

In general, you should not have to pay to participate in a clinical trial and you should be allowed to withdraw from the study at any time if you so choose. Many clinical trials offer minimal payment to participants. The only costs you generally have with clinical studies are transportation costs, if you have to travel to the site of the clinical trial.

Like the general public, you will learn the results of the clinical trial when it has concluded and researchers publish their findings.

Before enrolling in a clinical trial, you should ask as many questions from the study's coordinator as you can to ensure you feel safe and confident in participating. Do not be afraid to ask questions; even the National Institutes of Health encourage prospective participants to ask plenty of questions so they understand what to expect. You can learn more about the questions you should ask and about what to expect from clinical trials in general at the National Institutes of Health: http://www.nih.gov/health/clinicaltrials/basics.htm.

c. How to find Clinical Trials

Finding a clinical trial for which you may be eligible is easy. The government in the United States keeps track of all clinical trials that are currently recruiting at http://www.clinicaltrials.gov/. Go to the home page and in the search bar, type in "ALS" and click the search button.

You will then be presented with a list of current studies and their status, such as: Recruiting; Active, Not recruiting; Completed; Enrollment by invitation; Not yet recruiting; Terminated; and Unknown.

Click on the studies in which you are interested, and you will be able to read about the study, including the length of the study and the goals for the study, the eligibility requirements for you to participate in the study; and where in the country you must live to participate in the study. Contact information is available, so you can contact the researchers if you are interested in and eligible for a particular study.

You can also find a listing of ALS clinical trials through the Northeast Amyotrophic Lateral Sclerosis Consortium. The

ALS Association also funds research, which includes clinical trials.

Chapter Ten: Caregiver Tips

a. Affects of ALS on Loved Ones

A diagnosis of ALS does not just change the diagnosed individual's life. It changes the lives of family members and loved ones, especially those closest to the person with ALS. You will experience many of the same emotions as your loved one upon learning of their diagnosis: Anger, frustration, sadness, and grief. Many ALS patients and their loved ones go through the process of grieving upon learning of the diagnosis.

Allow yourself to go through whatever emotions you are experiencing and, if you are having difficulty with those emotions, do not be hesitant to reach out for help, whether by talking with a psychologist, a religious counselor, or someone who can effectively assist you in dealing with your feelings.

If you are going to be the caregiver for your loved one, your life is going to drastically change, but your life does not have to become unrecognizable. You can still maintain the sense of normality your family had before your loved one's diagnosis.

In this chapter, we are going to discuss you, the caregiver, and how you can make life easier for yourself and, in doing so, for your loved one.

b. What is a caregiver?

You have already read the term "caregiver" repeatedly throughout this book and you have probably heard it mentioned by doctors and other medical professionals. But, what does being a caregiver for your loved one really mean? What can you expect and how will you take care of yourself to ensure you remain physically and mentally healthy?

Your role as a caregiver for your loved one with ALS will evolve as your loved one's ALS progresses. What may start out as a small but significant role will eventually become more demanding.

In the beginning, your loved one may only need your assistance for simple things like helping to button a shirt and tying his shoes. As the ALS progresses, your loved one will depend more and more on you, and on any other caregivers, to help with feeding, dressing, bathing, and getting in and out of bed and so on.

Some people with ALS opt for a ventilator when breathing becomes difficult. A ventilator requires around the clock care from a registered nurse, a respiratory therapist, or another medical professional. Caregivers sometimes go through training to allow them to watch the ventilator and make sure it

is working properly. If your loved one decides to use a ventilator, are you willing to be trained so you can continue providing the necessary care? It is a question which you might want to start thinking about now, so you are prepared if the time comes and your loved one begins using a ventilator.

Caregivers are part of a team that includes medical professionals and the loved one with ALS. Your loved one with ALS will also be part of caring for himself, as long as he is able to do so. Encourage your loved one to do the things that can still be done for himself and make him feel part of the team.

Your loved one may become frustrated or angry that he cannot do things for himself anymore. That is normal. Remain patient with your loved one and assist when asked.

You, too, may become frustrated or angry at times. That is normal, too. Caregivers cannot do it alone. Instead of trying to do it alone, and facing eventual burnout which we will discuss in the next section, build a team of trusted family members and friends who are willing to help out, too. You will also have the support of other medical professionals, including your doctor, an occupational therapist, a physical therapist, or a counselor that can provide you with the skills that will help make managing your loved one's ALS easier.

c. Tips for Caring for Yourself whilst Caring for a Loved One

You may have not even given a second thought to whether or not you would become your loved one's caregiver when you heard the doctor say "ALS." Many people naturally step into the role of caregiver, often forgetting about themselves in the process.

As you go through your journey as a caregiver, keep the following tips in mind:

Take time for yourself

As a caregiver, you are going to be on-call 24 hours a day, 7 days a week. Your loved one is going to increasingly depend on you as their disease progresses, especially if your loved one will live at home for the remainder of their life. Caregivers often focus so much of their time and their energy on their loved one that they neglect themselves. Take time to care for yourself both physically and emotionally, so you avoid burnout and better care for your loved one.

Your loved one will express their needs to you, and you should do the same with them. Maintain friendships and continue with activities to allow some time for yourself. Perhaps before your loved one's diagnosis, you went out to dinner with your best friend every Thursday evening. Continue with that tradition, allowing another family member or friend to spend time with your loved one while you are out.

Do not feel selfish for taking care of yourself

Some caregivers feel selfish for wanting a break or needing to take time for themselves. You are not selfish for wanting and for needing to take time to yourself. If you do not care for yourself and for your emotional and physical needs, you are not going to be able to properly care for your loved one.

Become educated about ALS

Most people probably have heard about ALS, or Lou Gehrig's Disease, but unless they are directly affected by it or work with people with ALS, they most probably do not know much about it. Learn as much as you can about ALS, so you know what to expect from each stage of the disease and how you can help your loved one live as long and as comfortably as possible.

In addition to increasing your knowledge about ALS, learn about your role as a caregiver. What is generally expected of a caregiver with ALS? How can you avoid burnout? How can you make your loved one's life easier and better without losing yourself in the disease? A support group of caregivers can provide you with a sense of community and will allow you to forge friendships with others who know what you are going through.

You can find a list of valuable educational resources and links in Chapters Fifteen and Sixteen.

Know the Warning Signs of Depression

Sometimes the pressures of caring for a loved one with ALS can become too much. Depression is common among caregivers, but it is manageable through treatment such as counseling with a psychologist or another professional and medication or a combination of the two.

The Mayo Clinic cites several common signs of depression, including:

- You cry for no reason.

- You begin to have suicidal thoughts.

- You are tired and lack the energy you normally have; a simple task that should take a few minutes now takes much longer and requires all of your effort to complete.

- You have difficulty concentrating.

- You are not getting pleasure from everyday activities that you normally enjoy.

- You either cannot sleep or you sleep too much.

- Changes in your appetite. Some people with depression eat more than usual which causes weight gain while others find their appetite decreases, causing weight loss.

- You generally feel sad or have feelings of hopelessness.

- You begin to feel worthless or have feelings of guilt.

If you exhibit any of the symptoms of depression for two or more weeks, you may be suffering from clinical depression. Contact your doctor immediately to determine the best course of action to get you feeling better.

Identifying Caregiver Burnout

Sometimes caregivers become depressed because they are simply burned out. Burnout is a common problem among caregivers, regardless of the type of disease or illness their loved ones have. Burnout can have numerous different causes, such as:

- **Pressure.** You may feel pressure to be perfect, neglecting to appreciate all that you have accomplished as a caregiver for your loved one.

- **Pent up emotions.** You may be afraid to express how you really feel, allowing your emotions to build up inside of you.

- **Too much to do.** You may feel overwhelmed with how much you have to do every day. Sometimes, no matter how you look at it, there are not enough hours in the day.

- **Inability to separate your roles**. Many caregivers, especially in the beginning, have difficulty separating their role as a caregiver with their role as a spouse or a parent.

Symptoms of Burnout

You may start to feel the effects of burnout, which can manifest itself in one or more several common symptoms, such as:

- You may start to feel run down and begin developing headaches, fatigue, and general pain in your body. You may also have difficulty sleeping or you may feel lethargic, struggling to accomplish even the simplest of tasks.

- If you are normally a positive, cheerful person, you may start to feel overwhelmed by negative emotions – anger, frustration, and even guilt – that you just cannot shake.

- You may begin to overindulge in things that make you feel good, whether it is alcohol, cigarettes, food, or caffeine as a way of dealing with all that is going on or to calm your nerves.

- You feel as though you are on an emotional roller coaster; fine one minute and frustrated the next; back to normal then overwhelmed by anger.

- You begin to withdraw from your everyday life, avoiding friends and keeping your thoughts and your feelings to yourself.

- You begin avoiding activities that take you outside of your role as a caregiver. Maybe you go to church every Sunday or you are part of a group of friends that goes bowling every Tuesday night, and you no longer show up.

- You find yourself making excuses every time a family member or a loved one calls you and asks you to go out and spend time with him or her.

- You stop caring about how you look, whether it is no longer getting haircuts like you used to, buying new clothes, or having your nails done.

- You can no longer concentrate or function properly at work. Your mind may constantly be on your loved one, even when you are at work, and things you need to do for them. You may be forced to take time off of work to take care of your loved one.

- You may become forgetful, unintentionally missing scheduled appointments and forgetting birthdays, for

  example.

- You just do not feel like yourself.

Burnout is normal and common. If you are aware of the signs, you can avoid burnout or if burnout is unavoidable, you can work toward getting yourself rejuvenated and back to normal.

Tips for Avoiding Burnout

Expect periods of burnout during your time as a caregiver. You may be able to avoid long periods of burnout or recover from burnout in any number of ways. Following are several tips on how to avoid burning out.

Watch your diet

Eat a proper diet. Make sure you get enough proper nutrition each day. Even if you do not feel like eating, make sure you try to eat healthy foods and spread your meals out. Instead of eating three main meals a day, eat smaller meals throughout the day.

Avoid alcohol and tobacco

Avoid using alcohol or smoking, both of which could make you feel worse rather than better. Many people do not realize that alcohol actually works as a depressant, which slows down your nervous system. Alcohol generally enhances your feelings. If you have been feeling stressed and depressed, you may become even more depressed as a result of your alcohol consumption.

Remain active

Make time for physical activity, even if it is just a brisk walk around your neighborhood. Exercise has proven to help alleviate the symptoms of depression as well.

You may also want to try different stress relief techniques, such as meditation or yoga. Treat yourself to a massage that will allow both your body and your mind to relax and to rejuvenate.

Write

Consider writing in a journal. You may have feelings you do not want to share with anyone or you may just want to vent without feeling as though you will be judged. Journaling can be an effective and a cathartic way to deal with everything that is going on in your life.

Get sufficient sleep

Make sure you get enough sleep each night. Having a set sleep schedule helps ensure sufficient sleep. If possible, go to bed around the same time each night and wake up around the same time each morning. If you are tired during the day and if you can, take a nap.

Pet therapy

Spend time with a pet or around animals. Animals can have an extremely calming effect on people. Many pets – dogs, cats, and rabbits – are even trained as therapy pets to help people in stressful situations. After the bombings at the Boston Marathon in 2013, therapy dogs visited survivors in Boston's hospitals. If you have a pet, spend time with them. If you do not have a pet, consider volunteering an hour or two of your time at your local animal shelter. You may be surprised to find how calm you feel for that time, even if you feel as though you are living in the middle of a storm.

Delegate

Be realistic about how much you can do. Everyone has limits, and you can only accomplish so much in a 24 hour period.

Figure out what you can do and what you can delegate for others to do, so you do not become overwhelmed. Remember that it is okay to ask for help. Asking for help does not make you weak nor will family and friends think less of you for it.

Follow a routine

Establish and follow a daily routine. Knowing what you will do and when you will do it throughout the day will alleviate pressure and will allow you to get done what needs to be done. A routine also allows your loved to feel a sense of security, knowing that there is order to the day.

Listen to music

Music is a great way for some people to forget their troubles. A favorite singer or song may take you on a happy journey down memory lane with your loved one, which can help you rejuvenate. Music is often cathartic.

Be creative

Some people find that creative activities, such as drawing and painting, are an ideal way to relieve stress and to just enjoy the moment. You may enjoy crocheting, knitting, pottery, or any number of creative activities that allow you to relax.

Learn how to say no

You are only one person and you can only do so much. Learn how to say no to the things you do not have time to do or you simply do not want to do. On the flip side, allow yourself to say yes to activities you do enjoy, even if it means spending time away from your loved one.

Consult your doctor

If you are experiencing physical symptoms of burnout that linger, make an appointment with your doctor.

Know your priorities

Make a list of the responsibilities you have in your life and prioritize them. Knowing your priorities will help you ensure that you get done what needs to be done and that you are there for the people who matter the most in your life.

Surround yourself with positive people

You, like your loved one with ALS, are going to deal with your fair share of negative emotions. You are dealing with something most people do not understand. Surround yourself with family members and loved ones who will listen to you vent and who are generally positive overall.

Find balance

One of the biggest challenges any of us, but especially caregivers, face is learning how to balance all the responsibilities we have in life.

Remember, you are not just a caregiver to your loved one. If you are caring for a spouse with ALS, do not allow your role as caregiver to overtake your role as a husband or as a wife. Find ways to keep the romance alive, whether it is eating dinner by candlelight, watching a favorite movie together, or just sitting together and holding hands.

d. Finding and Accepting Care Giving Assistance

You are not alone in caring for your loved one. Many caregivers, however, feel a sense of obligation to their loved one to accept the responsibility for their care and have difficulty asking for and accepting assistance. Some caregivers feel as though, if they ask for help, they will be letting family and friends, who admire their strength and their role as caregiver, down in some way.

Start by building a team of trusted family members and friends who are willing to help with your loved one's care. You may be the person closest to your loved one, but as we just discussed you cannot do it all by yourself. You can try, but you will inevitably face burnout.

You can build your own care team, especially if you have family members and friends who want to help. The ALS Association of Philadelphia recommends choosing someone who is close to you to act as a coordinator. The coordinator should not be the primary caregiver as the primary caregiver already has enough to do.

The coordinator will then be responsible for delegating tasks, such as cooking and doing the laundry, with those who have offered to help. The ALS Association of Philadelphia recommends providing the coordinator with two lists. The first list should define all of the tasks with which you may need help, from laundry to taking your dog for a walk, and may even include helping to care for your loved one. The second list should consist of all of those people who have offered to help and their contact information.

The coordinator will then be responsible for contacting those people who have offered to help and asking if they will complete certain tasks. You will always know what is going on as the coordinator will create a calendar, listing who will be completing what tasks and the date and the approximate time those tasks will be completed.

Asking for help can be difficult, especially if you are the kind of person who does not generally ask for it. But, by building a caregiver team, you can ensure that all of the necessary tasks are completed and you will have more time to care for your loved one. Just as importantly, you will have the time you need to take care of yourself so you can be there for your loved one.

e. Support: Connecting with Other ALS families

A select group of people understand exactly what you, your loved one, and your family are going through as you adapt to a life that includes ALS: Other ALS families. Support groups can be an effective way of dealing with the many emotional, physical, and other issues you and your loved one will now face as a result of ALS.

Talk with your medical support team (doctor, occupational therapist, speech pathologist, physical therapist, and social worker) to see if they can recommend a local support group. Many hospitals also keep lists of support groups available to those with ALS.

You can find support groups in your area by visiting the ALS Association Chapter Support Groups at http://www.alsa.org/community/support-groups/.

Chapter Eleven: Planning for End of Life

An ALS diagnosis gives no indication of how long a patient will survive. You could live the median range of 2 to 5 years or enjoy another 20 or 30 years. You just do not know, which makes planning for the end of life even more important.

Once you and your loved ones have come to terms with your diagnosis, you should begin thinking about the legal and the practical aspects of the end of life to ensure your wishes are heard and are respected. Discuss such issues with your closest family members, and when necessary, seek legal counsels.

Make the decisions that are best for you and are what you want, and make sure you tell your family members what you have ultimately decided so they can respect and, if necessary, adhere to your wishes.

a. Living Will

A living will allows you to control what will happen to you in case you are incapacitated and cannot make decisions for yourself. Your living will defines what you want to happen if lifesaving measures, such as a feeding tube, are necessary to continue living.

In your living will, you will stipulate what lifesaving measures you want and which you do not want. For example, you may not want CPR to revive you if you stop breathing or your heart stops, but you may decide that you want a feeding tube to sustain you if you are no longer able to eat on your own.

To ensure you comply with the laws in your state, consider consulting with an attorney to determine what needs to be done to make sure your living will is valid. Generally, however, you will be required to have your living will certified by your doctor.

A living will is not set in stone. You can make changes to it at any time, as long as you are of sound mind.

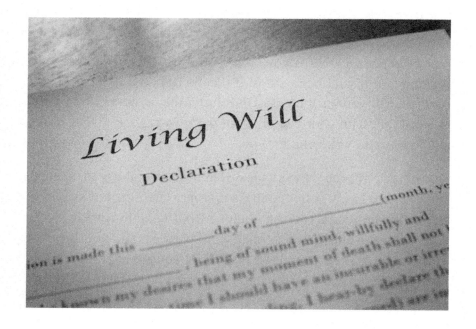

b. Do Not Resuscitate (DNR)

A Do Not Resuscitate, or DNR, order allows you to choose not to have lifesaving measures taken to revive you if you stop breathing or your heart stops beating. If you choose a DNR and you stop breathing, medical professionals cannot go against your wishes and cannot perform CPR, electric heart shock, chest compressions, or any of the lifesaving methods designated to save your life.

You only need a DNR if you do not want CPR if you stop breathing or if your heart stops. If you do not want to be resuscitated, you must have a DNR order that is written by your doctor. Talk with your doctor about your wishes for a DNR order and ask him to write one for you.

How the DNR process works is different from country to country, so be sure to know your country's or your state's requirements. Generally, however, you can obtain a DNR card, to carry with you or to keep at home, or a bracelet to wear, should you stop breathing or should your heart stop while you are at home. The DNR order will also be included in your medical chart, so doctors know not to use CPR or any other methods that will prolong your life.

Your DNR wishes should be specified in your living will, if you have one, and you should make sure your loved ones, and the person who has power of attorney for you, knows and will abide by your request should the time come and the DNR need to be enforced.

You can learn more about DNR orders from the National Institutes of Health and the U.S. National Library of Medicine at http://www.nlm.nih.gov/medlineplus/ency/patientinstructions/000 473.htm.

c. Choosing a Health Agent

You may not always be in the position to make your own decisions, especially as your disease progresses. Appointing a health care agent will allow someone you trust to make decisions on your behalf. If you are unable to speak and the doctors want to put you on life support, your health agent can tell them not to because it goes against your wishes or vice-versa. If the doctor wants to perform a surgery and your agent knows it is not something you want, he can refuse on your behalf.

Your health care agent will make decisions for you based on what you and he/she have discussed about what you want and do not want based on what you have stated in your living will. A health care agent makes sure doctors, and others, adhere to your wishes, despite their personal feelings.

Deciding who should be your health agent is important and can be difficult. You must find someone who knows what you want in terms of end of life care and lifesaving measures and who, most importantly, will respect your wishes and do what you would want.

When considering who should be your health agent, really consider whether that person has the ability to make clear, rational decisions that will be in your best interests and in accordance with what you want. Talk with the person at great length about what you want, and make sure they are emotionally willing to make decisions on your behalf, no matter how difficult those decisions may be. If you do not want to be kept on life support, will your health agent be able to tell the doctors to remove you from it? Ask hard questions before choosing a health agent.

You do not have to choose a family member to represent you. Consider whether a family member would have a difficult time adhering to your wishes of enforcing a DNR, for example, because he or she does not want to lose you.

Do not allow others to influence you into choosing them to represent you and do not choose an individual because you feel obligated to do so or because you would feel guilty if you did not choose that person.

Whoever you choose as a health agent, you must make your choice official by filling out a medical power of attorney form, which you can generally obtain from any attorney's office or from your local hospital. You can legally request a change of your health agent at any time, provided you are considered to be of sound mind.

d. Power of Attorney

As ALS progresses, you may deal with dementia or be faced with other issues that make it impossible for you to make decisions about your health or your finances any longer. As we just discussed, a designated health agent can make medical decisions on your behalf. A power of attorney can make

financial and legal decisions on your behalf and can legally sign checks on your behalf, can file your taxes for you, can run your business (if applicable), and can handle any real estate you own.

Generally, the health agent (medical power of attorney) and individual with power of attorney are two different individuals to avoid any potential conflict of interest.

e. Hospice Care

As your ALS progresses and you may need around the clock care, do you want to seek hospice care? Hospice care typically occurs in the home, although it may be available if you are in a nursing facility or in the hospital. Many hospices also offer a hospice house into which individuals at the end of life can move for around the clock care. If the hospice with which you are working does not have a hospice house, talk with the lead doctor or social worker who may be able to find a hospice house for you.

A hospice house is designed to be like your own house and to ensure your comfort and the comfort of family. If you move into a hospice house, you will be cared for by nurses and a staff of medical professionals in addition to your regular doctors.

Hospice care is headed by a doctor who leads a team of caregivers, including nurses, social workers, and home health aides. The team works together to determine the best treatment and care plan so you will be comfortable in the end stages of ALS. Nurses are generally available, when needed, around the clock, while home health aides can assist caregivers in caring for their loved one, giving them a much needed break. Social workers generally help the ALS patient and family members with the many emotions that abound at the end of life.

Volunteers also work with hospices and often visit ALS patients and their families to help with tasks that are not medical related. A volunteer may assist you in completing tasks and will allow you to enjoy conversation with a friendly, understanding individual.

Individuals are generally eligible for hospice care if doctors believe they have six months or less to live. Hospice care is also designed for those individuals who want to spend the remainder of their lives comfortable and cared for but who no longer want to try new treatments to prolong their lifespan. You may, for example, be on a ventilator to help you breathe, but you want to stop using the ventilator. You will probably be eligible for hospice care.

Americans with Medicare or Medicaid are normally covered for hospice care, while many insurance plans will only cover hospice care if the patient has a life expectancy of less than six months.

f. Planning Your or Your Loved One's Funeral

Some people prefer to plan their own funeral prior to their death. If you want to determine how your life is celebrated after you are gone, talk with your family about your funeral and start making arrangements now. If you are a caregiver, you may want to wait until your loved one begins to talk about dying before you gently broach the subject of a funeral or a memorial service.

Your loved one may not want to be involved in the planning of their funeral. If that is the case, pay attention when you are talking with them, as they may talk about information, such as a favorite song, you can use during funeral arrangements. Perhaps they have always said they wanted to be cremated rather than buried or buried in a mausoleum rather than in a traditional grave. Listen for what your loved one has to say, so you can give them what they want when they're gone.

Some people with terminal illnesses opt to have a celebration of life before they pass away, which can allow them to enjoy time with family and friends, all at the same time, while celebrating the life they had together. Others prefer to plan for the memorial service after they are gone. Your loved one may prefer that people remember them and be happy, celebrating life with a party. You and your loved one may want to work together to create a video or photographic collage of your lives together, which you can then play during the memorial service.

Planning for a funeral is a very personal and difficult task, and the most important thing to remember is to follow your loved one's lead. If they want to talk about and to plan for the memorial service, do so together. If they do not, that is perfectly fine, too, and it is something you can think about as the time nears.

g. Donating To ALS Research

Organ donation is not always possible with ALS due to the ravages of the disease on some of the body's organs. If you are interested in donating your organs, make sure you are listed as an organ donor or at the very least make sure your doctor is made aware of your wish to donate your organs. Whether your organs can be donated upon your death really depends on the state of your organs at the time of death. The doctors at the hospital who harvest your organs will make the final determination.

If you are not sure about organ donation or if you have questions about how it works, talk with your doctor. Your doctor can answer any questions you may have, which will allow you to make a final decision with which you are comfortable.

The decision to be or not to be an organ donor is not a permanent one and you can change your mind at any time, provided you make sure medical professionals and your loved ones are aware of your decision.

You can learn more about donating your organs and organ donation in general at the U.S. Department of Health and Human Service's orgondonor.gov: http://www.organdonor.gov/index.html.

Some people with ALS have decided to donate their bodies to ALS research, which can provide valuable evidence into the inner workings of the disease. A donation of your body to ALS research will allow researchers to, according to Massachusetts General Hospital, study the nerves in your brain and in your spinal cord, which is difficult to do when a patient is alive.

Massachusetts General Hospital offers a list of those facilities in the United States that accept body and tissue donations from those who have passed away from ALS. To access the full list, go to http://www.massgeneral.org/als/assets/pdf/fyi_tissue.pdf.

h. Keep Good Records

You may feel somewhat overwhelmed by all of the decisions you and your loved ones must make. The best way to keep track of what is going on and the decisions your loved one has made about current and future care is to keep good records of all legal information. Choose a recordkeeping system, such as file folders, that works best for you and maintain information such as:

- A copy of the will, the living will, and the DNR order, (if applicable).

- A record of your medical power of attorney and of your power of attorney.

- Life insurance policies.

- The deed to the home.

You will also need to keep records of your loved one's medical information, keeping it in an easy to access place, so you can grab it and take it with you if you need to rush to the hospital or to the doctor's office. Such information should include:

- A list of emergency contacts and their contact information.

- All of the doctors your loved one sees and their contact information.

- A list of caregivers – such as occupational therapist, respiratory therapist, speech pathologist, and physical therapist – and their contact information.

- A list of medications, including the dosage and how often your loved one takes the medication.

- A list of allergies, if applicable, to medications.

- A copy of your health insurance card, and if you do not have a copy of your card, all of the necessary information you may need, including your insurance carrier and your account number.

- The ALS patient's blood type.

- A history of the patient's care, including a list of appointments, dates and reasons for any hospitalizations, and treatment.

- A list of assistive equipment, such as a walker or a breathing mask, currently being used.

- A description of any special needs or issues with care.

Keep all of your records together so you can just grab them when you need them. If something happens to you and another caregiver needs to take over in an emergency, that caregiver will have all of the information they need to properly care for your loved one.

Chapter Twelve: Famous People with ALS

Amyotrophic Lateral Sclerosis has become better known today, in part because of the power of the media and the celebrities who often give a face to the progressive neuromuscular disease.

a. Lou Gehrig

Lou Gehrig, who we already discussed in the introduction, is perhaps one of history's most famous people with ALS. The famed first baseman for the New York Yankees was perhaps best known for the grace with which he played the game and his impressive 2,130 consecutive games played streak, which only ended when the early symptoms of ALS affected his ability to play. He removed himself from the Yankees' starting lineup for the first time in 14 years in May of 1939. Gehrig would die two years later on June 2, 1941. Gehrig's prominence at the time of his diagnosis resulted in many people, from then on, referring to ALS as Lou Gehrig's Disease.

b. Stephen Hawking

Stephen Hawking is, aside from Lou Gehrig, perhaps the best known person with ALS in the world. Hawking was diagnosed with ALS at the age of 21, more than five decades ago, in 1963. After his diagnosis, the British-born Hawking married and continued on with his studies and his eventual work as a scientist, earning a doctorate and becoming one of the world's most celebrated physicists and lecturers. He is the best-selling author of such works as "A Brief History of Time," "A Briefer History of Time," and "The Universe in a Nutshell." His latest book is "The

Grand Design." To learn more about Stephen Hawking, his career, and his five decade long victory against ALS, check out his official website at http://www.hawking.org.uk/.

c. Jason Becker

Jason Becker gained fame as a metal guitarist with David Lee Roth's band. But, after recording a single album with Roth, Becker's life and career took a sharp turn. The then 19 year old musician was diagnosed with Lou Gehrig's Disease. Becker would, like many ALS patients, lose his ability to speak. Still, he continues to communicate using an assistive device and he

still composes music. A film about his battle with ALS, "Jason Becker: Not Dead Yet," was released to critical acclaim in 2012. To learn more about Jason Becker's 20 year battle against ALS, check out his website at: http://jasonbeckerguitar.com/jasons_words.html.

d. Huddie William Ledbetter

Huddie William Ledbetter, or better known as Lead Belly, was one of America's leading folk and blues singers in the early part of the 20th century. His career was almost sidetracked, however, when in 1918 he received a 30 year prison sentence for killing a man with whom he had gotten into a fight. The governor of Texas pardoned Lead Belly in 1925, after the musician wrote him a song asking to be pardoned. Ledbetter would go on to become a famous folk musician with such songs as "Goodnight Irene" and "Midnight Special." The folk musician was diagnosed with ALS in the 1940s, losing his battle with the disease in 1949 at the age of 64 or 68 (records varied as to whether he was born in 1885 or 1889).

e. Charles Mingus

American jazz musician Charles Mingus is perhaps best known for his piece, "Goodbye, Porkiepie Hat," which musicians continue to remake. He also released numerous albums, including "Mingus Ah Um," "Blues and Roots," and "The Black Saint and the Sinner Lady." The Mingus Awareness Project periodically holds musical events to raise funds for the awareness of and to provide support for those with ALS and their families. Charles Mingus died from ALS on January 5, 1979 at the age of 57.

f. David Niven

British-born actor David Niven is perhaps best known for his portrayal of Phileas Fogg in the film "Around the World in Eighty Days" and as Sir Charles Lytton in "The Pink Panther." Niven earned the highest of Hollywood owners when he won an Academy Award for the 1958 film "Separate Tables." Niven was diagnosed with Lou Gehrig's Disease in 1981 and died only two years later on July 29, 1983. He was 73.

g. Morrie Schwartz

Morrie Schwartz's battle with ALS became well-known in mainstream American, due to Mitch Albom's memoir "Tuesdays with Morrie." Schwarz was a professor at Brandeis University. He lost his battle with ALS on November 4, 1995 at the age of 79.

h. Lane Smith

American actor Lane Smith, perhaps most famous for his portrayal of Perry White in the television show "Lois & Clark," starred on both TV and the silver screen, appearing in such television shows as "The Practice," "Judging Amy," and the animated "King of the Hill," and in films such as "The Legend of Bagger Vance," "My Cousin Vinny," and "The Mighty Ducks." Smith, whose career dated back to 1966, lost his battle with ALS on June 13, 2005. He was 69.

i. Michael Zaslow

Most American soap opera fans, regardless of their favorite soap, have undoubtedly heard of the Michael Zaslow, who starred on both Guiding Light and One Life to Live throughout his career. Zaslow played the villain Roger Thorpe on Guiding Light for 25 years, losing his job in early 1997, only eight months after his speech became slurred, according to The New York Times. Zaslow was diagnosed with ALS later in 1997 and immediately became a face of Lou Gehrig's Disease. In his effort to educate the public about ALS, Zaslow returned to One Life to Live as David Renaldi, a pianist who was now facing the life or death struggles of Lou Gehrig's Disease. Zaslow died a year after his diagnosis at age 56 on December 6, 1998.

j. Mao Zedong

Mao Zedong, who is credited with founding the People's Republic of China, is described as a revolutionary warrior and is most commonly referred to as Chairman Mao. Mao died in September of 1976, at the age of 82, from complications of ALS.

k. Other Famous People with ALS

- Jeff Julian (Golfer)
- Glenn Montgomery (Football player)
- Bruce Edwards (PGA golf caddy)
- Jim "Catfish" Hunter (Baseball player)
- Dmitri Shostakovich (Russian composer)
- Jacob Javitz (U.S. senator)
- Orlando Thomas (Football player)
- Charlie Wedemeyer (High school teacher and football coach)

Chapter Thirteen: Hope for a Cure: Developments in Research

Researchers have been working to find out the exact cause of ALS and how to effectively treat and cure it for decades. Research is ongoing, with researchers consistently making new discoveries, including the prospective benefits of stem cell transplants, identifying two genes that appear in approximately 40 percent of all familial ALS cases, and studying whether damaged protein found in those with ALS can be treated with medication to reverse the affects of and to eventually cure Lou Gehrig's Disease.

a. Stem Cell Research

For the past decade, researchers in multiple institutions throughout the United States have been studying the effect of transplanted stem cells in individuals with Lou Gehrig's Disease. Remember, ALS destroys the nerves in the spinal cord, resulting in muscle weakness and in respiratory problems in people with ALS.

What researchers found, according to an article published by the Harvard Medical School, was when healthy stem cells were transplanted into mice with familial ALS, the progression of the disease began to slow down and the mice began having an easier time breathing. In fact, the mice that received transplanted stem cells lived between three and four times longer than the mice that did not receive the stem cell transplants.

Healthy stem cells for the transplant can be used from adults, including from the individual with ALS. Using an individual's stem cells offers several benefits. Because the stem cells are from the individual's own body, they should not experience any negative effects. In addition, controversy surrounds the process of using embryonic stem cells and using an individual's own stems cells removes the controversy and stress from the process for those involved.

Researchers caution that the discovery of the benefits of stem cell transplants is not a cure, but it may help slow the progression of the disease and may increase the life expectancy in individuals with ALS, as it did in the mice used as models.

To learn more about the researchers' findings, visit the Harvard Medical School at http://hms.harvard.edu/news/treatment-als-1-2-13.

A summary of the studies conducted by researchers from various institutions, including Johns Hopkins University and Columbia University, was published in Science Transitional Magazine, which can be viewed by going to: http://stm.sciencemag.org/content/4/165/165ra164.

b. Genetic Research

Researchers at St. Jude's Children's Research Hospital announced in March of 2013 that they have identified two genes with mutations that result in the death of nerve cells in those individuals with Lou Gehrig's Disease. The mutation in both genes results from an abundance of protein accumulating inside the body's cells. The result is damaged protein, which we will discuss in the next section, which does not allow the body's RNA to function properly.

Researchers believe that the mutated genes and damaged protein may be a common cause in ALS, cancer, and other neuromuscular diseases and that the newly discovered information may allow researchers to develop treatments that could help fix the gene mutation and damaged proteins.

c. Damaged Protein

Researchers at Northwestern University announced the findings of a study in 2011 citing the possible connection between damaged proteins and Lou Gehrig's Disease. The damaged protein ubiquilin 2, according to researchers, has been found in both sporadic and familial instances of ALS.

The damaged proteins build up in the neurons of the spinal cord and of the brain in people with ALS. That build up of damaged proteins hinders the proper functioning of the nervous system, making it difficult for the nerves to send signals to the body. As a result, people with ALS begin to lose the ability to breathe and to swallow properly.

Researchers, according to reports, can now conduct studies to find out if conventional medication already on the market may help in fixing the damaged protein so it can work properly in those with ALS.

Chapter Fourteen: ALS Resources & Organizations in the USA

1. ALS Association
   http://www.alsa.org/

2. ALS Les Turner Foundation of Chicago
   http://www.lesturnerals.org/

3. ALS Worldwide
   http://www.alsworldwide.org/

4. National Amyotrophic Lateral Sclerosis Registry
   http://wwwn.cdc.gov/als/

5. ALS Therapy Development Institute
   http://www.als.net/

6. ALS Therapy Alliance
   http://alstherapyalliance.org/index.php

7. Project ALS
   http://www.projectals.org/index.html

8. The Robert Packard Center for ALS Research at Johns Hopkins
   http://www.alscenter.org/

9. International Alliance of ALS/MND Associations
   http://www.alsmndalliance.org/

10. ALS Hope Foundation

http://www.alshopefoundation.org/

11. Prize4Life
    http://www.prize4life.org/

12. Muscular Dystrophy ALS Division
    http://als-mda.org/disease/amyotrophic-lateral-sclerosis

13. Northeast ALS Consortium (NEALS)
    http://www.alsconsortium.org/

14. ALS Clinical Trials
    http://www.clinicaltrials.gov/ct2/results?term=amyotrophi c+lateral+sclerosis

15. Emory ALS Center
    http://neurology.emory.edu/ALS/index.html

16. Compassionate Care ALS
    http://www.ccals.org/home.php

17. ALS Forums
    http://www.alsforums.com/

18. ALS Untangled
    http://www.alsuntangled.com/index.html

19. Familial ALS Registry
    https://fals.patientcrossroads.org/

20. National Institute of Neurological Disorders and Stroke

http://www.ninds.nih.gov/disorders/amyotrophiclateralscl
erosis/ALS.htm

21. Charlie Wedemeyer Family Outreach
    http://www.cwfo.org/alsinfo.html#learn

22. MDA/ALS Newsmagazine
    http://alsn.mda.org/

23. ALS Research Collaboration
    http://www.als-research.org/about/index.html

24. Duke ALS Clinic
    http://www.dukealsclinic.com/

25. The Mingus Awareness Project
    http://www.mingusawarenessproject.org/

26. ALS NeuroTalk Online Support Group
    http://neurotalk.psychcentral.com/forum6.html

27. The ALS Promise
    http://www.alspromise.org/

28. The ALS Guardian Angels
    http://www.alsguardianangels.com/

29. The ALS Recovery Fund
    http://www.alsrecovery.org/

30. The Peggy and Bernie Project
    http://www.peggyandbernieproject.org/about/

31. The War on ALS: Blazeman Foundation for ALS
    http://www.waronals.com/

32. The Busby Foundation
    http://www.busbyals.org/

33. The Johns Hopkins ALS Clinic
    http://www.hopkinsmedicine.org/neurology_neurosurgery
    /specialty_areas/als/

34. Massachusetts General Hospital ALS Multidisciplinary
    Clinic
    http://www.massgeneral.org/als/

35. Wake Forest Baptist Health ALS Clinic
    http://www.wakehealth.edu/Neurosciences/ALS/

36. A Treatment for ALS? Neural Stem Cell Transplants Slow
    Progression of Disease (Harvard Science)
    http://news.harvard.edu/gazette/story/2013/01/a-treatment-
    for-als/

37. Adult Stem Cells Tested to Treat ALS (Lou Gehrig's
    Disease) (LifeNews.com)
    http://www.lifenews.com/2011/09/21/adult-stem-cells-
    tested-to-treat-als-lou-gehrigs-disease/

38. Some hope seen in fight to cure ALS (Chicago Tribune)
    http://articles.chicagotribune.com/2013-03-20/news/ct-x-
    0320-expert-als-20130320_1_motor-neurons-als-cell-
    therapy

39. Two New Genes Linked to Amyotrophic Lateral Sclerosis (ALS) and Related Disorders (Science Daily) http://www.sciencedaily.com/releases/2013/03/130303154 857.htm

40. Study finds pathway to ALS cure (ABC7 Chicago) http://abclocal.go.com/wls/story?section=news/health&id =8320623

Chapter Fifteen: Other ALS Resources

a. United Kingdom

1. Motor Neuron Disease Association (MNDA) (The only organization in the United Kingdom that focuses on those with motor neuron diseases, like ALS, and their families). http://www.mndassociation.org/

2. ALS Genetic Mutation Database http://alsod.iop.kcl.ac.uk/

3. International Alliance of ALS/MND Associations http://www.alsmndalliance.org/

4. Patient.co.uk: ALS http://www.patient.co.uk/health/Motor-Neurone-Disease.htm

5. UCL Institute of Neurology & The National Hospital for Neurology and Neurosurgery http://www.ucl.ac.uk/ion/library/patient-info/a-z/a-b/amyotrophic

b. Canada

1. ALS Canada http://www.als.ca/

2. Robarts Research http://www.robarts.ca/als

3. Canadian ALS Research Network
   http://www.alsnetwork.ca/

4. ALS Society of British Columbia
   http://www.alsbc.ca/

5. Bombardier Plane Pull for ALS
   http://www.alsplanepull.ca/

6. ALS Society of Nova Scotia
   http://www.alsns.ca/

7. The ALS Clinic at the University of Alberta
   http://www.ualberta.ca/ALS/
8. ALS Canada on Twitter
   https://twitter.com/ALSCanada

9. The Derek Walton ALS Fund
   http://www.waltoncure4als.ca/

10. Help End ALS
    http://www.helpendals.ca/

c. **Australia**

1. MND Australia
   http://www.mndaust.asn.au/

2. Neuroscience Research Australia
   http://www.neura.edu.au/health/motor-neurone-disease-mnd

3. Genetic Support Council of Australia
    http://www.geneticsupportcouncil.org.au/conditions/view/lou-gehrigs-disease/
4. Motor Neuron Disease Association of WA
    http://www.mndawa.asn.au/

References

1. The ALS Association
   http://www.alsa.org/

2. National Institute of Neurological Disorders and Stroke –
   ALS Fact Sheet
   http://www.ninds.nih.gov/disorders/amyotrophiclateralscl
   erosis/detail_ALS.htm

3. UC San Diego Center for ALS Research and Therapy
   http://als.ucsd.edu/about-als/Pages/incidence.aspx

4. Johns Hopkins Medicine
   http://www.hopkinsmedicine.org/neurology_neurosurgery
   /specialty_areas/als/conditions/als_amyotrophic_lateral_sc
   lerosis.html

5. Mayo Clinic
   http://www.mayoclinic.com/health/amyotrophic-lateral-
   sclerosis/DS00359/DSECTION=causes

6. New York Yankees
   http://newyork.yankees.mlb.com/nyy/history/gehrig.jsp

7. Lou Gehrig's Speech from Sports Illustrated
   http://sportsillustrated.cnn.com/2009/baseball/mlb/07/04/g
   ehrig.text/index.html#ixzz2SGH41ynM

8. Muscular Dystrophy Association (Guamanian strain of
   ALS)

http://static.mda.org/research/020401batsALS.html

9. El Escorial Criteria for the Diagnosis of Amyotrophic
    Lateral Sclerosis (ALS)
    http://www.medicalcriteria.com/site/index.php?option=co
    m_content&view=article&id=54%3Aneuroals&catid=64
    %3Aneurology&Itemid=80&lang=en

10. Brain: A Journal of Neurology
    http://brain.oxfordjournals.org/content/early/2012/01/17/b
    rain.awr351.full

11. Muscular Dystrophy Association Classification System
    http://mda.org/disease/amyotrophic-lateral-sclerosis/signs-
    and-symptoms/stages-of-als

12. Emory University
    http://med.emory.edu/ADRC/dementias/frontotemporal_d
    ementia/

13. Nuedexta
    https://www.nuedexta.com/about-nuedexta/how-nuedexta-
    works

14. Rilutek – Mayo Clinic
    http://www.mayoclinic.com/health/amyotrophic-lateral-
    sclerosis/DS00359/DSECTION=treatments-and-drugs

15. Rilutek Side Effects – Web MD
    http://www.webmd.com/drugs/drug-12146-
    rilutek+oral.aspx?drugid=12146&drugname=rilutek+oral

16. Rilutek – ALS Association
    http://web.alsa.org/site/PageServer?pagename=ALSA_Ask_Dec2011

17. Massachusetts General Hospital
    http://www.massgeneral.org/als/patienteducation/depressionanxiety_ALS.aspx

18. Dartmouth Counseling and Human Development
    http://www.dartmouth.edu/~chd/resources/depression

19. ALS Association of Michigan
    http://www.alsofmi.org/

20. American Physical Therapy Association:
    http://www.apta.org/apta/findapt/index.aspx?navID=10737422525

21. Les Turner ALS Foundation
    http://www.lesturnerals.org/

22. Low Tech Solutions
    http://store.lowtechsolutions.org/

23. Model Talker
    http://www.modeltalker.com/

24. The ALS Association of Philadelphia
    http://www.alsphiladelphia.org/page.aspx?pid=934

25. ALS Association Community Chapters
    http://www.alsa.org/community/chapters/

26. The ALS Research Group
    http://www.alsrg.org/AlternativeTherapiesforALSPPT.pdf
    .pdf

27. Life Alert
    http://www.lifealert.com/

28. Dragon Speech Recognition Software
    http://www.nuance.com/dragon/index.htm

29. Medicaid
    http://www.medicaid.gov

30. Medicare
    http://www.medicare.gov/what-medicare-covers/

31. ALS Association of St. Louis
    http://webstl.alsa.org/site/PageServer?pagename=STL_ho
    mepage

32. National Institutes of Health (Clinical Trials)
    http://www.nichd.nih.gov/health/clinicalresearch/Pages/in
    dex.aspx

33. Northeast Amyotrophic Lateral Sclerosis Consortium
    http://www.alsconsortium.org/search.php

34. Organ Donation
    http://www.organdonor.gov/index.htm

35. Tissue and Body Donation
    http://www.massgeneral.org/als/assets/pdf/fyi_tissue.pdf

36. Jason Becker Not Dead Yet
    http://www.massgeneral.org/als/assets/pdf/fyi_tissue.pdf

37. Huddie Ledbetter
    http://www.songwritershalloffame.org/index.php/exhibits/
    bio/C16

38. Lead Belly Foundation
    http://www.leadbelly.org/re-homepage.html

39. The Mingus Awareness Project
    http://www.mingusawarenessproject.org/

40. Charles Mingus Official Website
    http://mingusmingusmingus.com

41. David Niven
    http://www.imdb.com/name/nm0000057/bio

42. Morrie Schwartz
    http://mitchalbom.com/d/bio/3720/inspiration-morrie-
    schwartz

43. Lane Smith
    http://www.imdb.com/name/nm0809031/

44. Michael Zaslow
    http://www.imdb.com/name/nm0953651/

45. Michael Zaslow – New York Times
    http://www.nytimes.com/1998/12/09/arts/michael-zaslow-

54-soap-actor-publicized-lou-gehrig-s-disease.html

46. Harvard Medical School
    http://hms.harvard.edu/news/treatment-als-1-2-13

47. St. Jude's Children's Research Hospital Study
    http://www.stjude.org/stjude/v/index.jsp?vgnextoid=bb2e
    89d1d5d1d310VgnVCM100000290115acRCRD&vgnext
    channel=2e2c338b30b6b310VgnVCM100000290115acR
    CRD&SearchUrl=search_results.jsp&QueryText=als%20s
    tudy

48. Nature, the International Journal of Science
    http://www.nature.com/nature/journal/v477/n7363/full/nat
    ure10353.html.

CPSIA information can be obtained at www.ICGtesting.com
Printed in the USA
BVOW06s1640230616

453027BV00008B/104/P